Volume 4, *POWER FOR DELIVERANCE SERIES*:

DELIVERANCE

FROM

CHILDLESSNESS

D1569002

BILL BANKS

Cover Design
SPB Studios

Special Thanks to
Camera Angle

Deliverance From Childlessness
ISBN 0-89228-0379

Copyright @ 1990
IMPACT BOOKS, INC.
137 W. Jefferson, Kirkwood, Mo. 63122
Printed in United States of America

Scripture quotations are from the Authorized King James Version, unless otherwise indicated.

FOREWORD

Although I have been engaged in medical practice as an obstetrician/gynecologist for nearly thirty years, and have worked with infertile couples on numerous occasions, sometimes having had our labors crowned with success and sometimes not, I had never truly considered infertility as possibly being the result of the presence of an evil spirit.

There were patients in whom tangible physical problems in the husband or wife were discovered and treated, with pregnancy resulting. There were other cases which did not respond to treatment and the couple remained infertile. In some instances even though insurmountable conditions were present, pregnancy unexpectedly occurred in response to prayer.

However, another category of couples was those in which no abnormalities could be found in either the husband or the wife. In many of these couples pregnancy would sometimes occur after many months or even years. But there were always those patients in whom pregnancy did not take place and it is this group, possibly who might most benefit from the ministry addressed in this book.

I have been privileged to know Bill Banks for fifteen years or more, and consider him both a friend and brother, and have learned from his previous writings, particularly *Ministering To*

Abortion's Aftermath. I have only seen a portion of the material in this book, but my appetite has been stimulated to see the entire manuscript.

Regardless of the way in which pregnancy occurs for the infertile couples whether by medical treatment, prayer, or spiritual warfare - to God be the glory for the victories though our Lord Jesus Christ!

Paul Ritter, M.D.
St. Louis, Mo.

TABLE OF CONTENTS

AUTHOR'S INTRODUCTION

THE MIRACLE OF CONCEPTION

Perhaps the real miracle is, that human conception ever occurs at all. The healthy male of the species regularly produces hundreds of millions of sperm each month, and if only one ultimately finds its' mark, it is sufficient to cause pregnancy. So, at best, the odds are millions to one against conception ever occurring even with two normally healthy individuals.

I will readily admit that the cases presented and described in this book do have what may be six areas of potential bias, because 1.) I am only relating cases with which I am personally familiar; 2.) they concern individuals with whom I have personally prayed. Honesty further necessitates that we observe that biases may be present due to the fact that the individuals 3.) were willing to seek prayer 4.) were willing to accept or acknowledge the sinfulness of certain activities and to repent of them (such as abortion, or pornography), and 5.) they all had at least a grain of faith to believe that God through prayer might intervene in their behalf and answer their prayers, which presupposes a belief that God exists and has such power. Additionally, 6.) the individuals in these studies have obviously had soft, repentant hearts; hearts submitted unto God, and were willing and eager to receive His ministry.

In my naivete, I assumed this problem of infertility or sterility to be primarily an American problem, but I've since discovered it to be both universal in scope, and not to be bounded by time. It crosses the centuries. I've also learned that the pain in the heart of an African mother denied a child, in an underdeveloped nation, is every bit as great as that experienced by the American suburbanite.

Many of us who have had some contact with the problem of infertility, also tend to think of it as a problem of relatively recent origin. It certainly is not. It has been around to some degree since the beginnings of recorded history, both biblical and secular.

The June 26, 1989 issue of *Insight Magazine*, carries an article, entitled "Penetrating Beyond The Pharaohs" which refers to discoveries made in Egyptian archaeological remains dating to fifth and sixth century Egypt. These came from a find in a small Egyptian town named Karanis, which is no longer in existence, and was located about a hundred miles south of present day Cairo.

In addition to the dramatic finds were also included the more mundane things of daily life. Found along with the other items were notes and letters handwritten by the common people of the time in Coptic (ancient Egyptian written in the Greek alphabet). Among them was found a copy of a prayer to be recited by a man in order for his wife to become pregnant.

Another interesting find in ancient Akhmim, in middle Egypt, was something that stretches across the fifteen hundred years, and reminds us of the powerful nature of curses. A curse was recorded that can be delivered against someone, against whom one has a grudge. It refers to an incantation to call upon the power of three angels, to cause the victim to experience "illness and rheum, and fever, and pain, and weariness, and depression, and chills, and tumors, and madness," and if that were not enough, "seventy different diseases." No doubt among those seventy were infertility and sterility. The curse closes with a statement that no other sorcerer or sorceress can erase it's power, save only the one who had placed it on the victim.

Since discovering many years ago while ministering to Charity, whose story is told in Part I, that both sterility and infertility can be spiritual in origin, and having seen God confirm this truth by causing "sterile couples" to produce offspring, and recognizing the immeasurable heart break and suffering caused by these two conditions, we have a desire to make available God's truth in bringing light to an area of darkness. We seek to share at least that portion of God's truth on the subject which has been revealed to us. The goal being to set captives free, to exalt Jesus, to expand His kingdom, to alleviate suffering, and to allow women previously denied children to have them.

The target for this book is mothers (desiring to be), those called upon to minister to mothers desiring-to-be, and to the body of Christ, that it might better understand the working of God's kingdom, and be the better equipped to offer loving compassion to hurting humanity.

Our prayer for you, if you are seeking children, is that you may, "Be fruitful and multiply ..."

And, if you are not seeking children, but instead a closer walk with Him, our prayer for you is similar, "Be fruitful in every good work." Also we pray that you might, as in John 15, *bear fruit, more fruit, much fruit*, and thus prove yourself to be His disciple.

If you wish it, may you truly find *Deliverance From Childlessness*!

PART I

A TENDER ISSUE

"Be fruitful, and multiply, and replenish the earth..."
(Gen. 1:28)

PART I

A TENDER ISSUE

The problem of infertility is extremely painful, not only for the woman, but for both partners in the marriage. The husband hurts just as does the wife over the absence of, or inability to have a child, plus he hurts for he is aware of the pain that his wife is experiencing. Each slight that she is confronted with pains him as well, because of his love for her.

Almost every woman is looking forward to the day when she can have a daughter to dress, and to teach to do things. Similarly, the potential father is looking forward to the day when he has a son of his own, with whom he can do things and share experiences.

Unfortunately the women without children are continually being reminded of their problem. They find painful reminders every time they open a woman's magazine and find articles concerning how to deal with children, teaching children, or how to nurture them. Every time such women are around friends who have children, and hear them mention their children, or their children's problems or successes, they are reminded of their own emptiness.

Similarly, every time there's a family function, and other members of the family are present with their children, they recall their own lack. A fresh hurt comes each time they learn of a friend or a relative who has become, or announced a preg-

7

nancy. The pain is reinforced. Especially painful are the unplanned pregnancies of acquaintances: "Why couldn't we who want a baby so badly have had that child, which they really don't even want or need?"

Satan loves to torment, and loves "to kick a woman when she's down." He can arrange to have the people ahead of her in a grocery market check out lane engage in discussing their babies, or expected additions. It seems as if everywhere the woman goes, daily experiences rub salt in the wound, enhancing the pain of her childlessness, as she attends functions and sees happy people with their children.

Tragically the couples faced with infertility very often find it difficult to communicate with one another about the issue, because of the tremendous pain that both experience. They find it easier not to even discuss it. Such problems place undue additional stress upon the marriage. Each time the words "child," "having a child," "pregnancy," "child bearing," or "fruitfulness" are heard by the infertile mother, the pain is like an arrow piercing her heart.

> "The horseleach hath two daughters, crying,
> Give, give. There are three things that are
> never satisfied, yea, four things say not, It is
> enough:
>
> "The grave; and the barren womb; the earth
> that is not filled with water; and the fire that
> saith not, It is enough." (Prov. 30:15,16)

These two verses from Proverbs describe four things that are never satisfied, the grave, barrenness, the desert needing water, and the burning of fire. The grave or death's desire for souls, the desert's thirsting desire for water, but having its all consuming desire never satisfied because it remains a desert and the burning flame that consumes all in its path. These are three descriptions paralleling the condition of childlessness.

8

The infertile couple experiences grief and loss over the unborn child they have not yet seen in much the way parents would who had lost a child through death whom they had seen. The difference being, that the infertile couple has never seen their child, never had the joy of playing with it, seeing its first smile, enjoying and sharing birthdays with it. But their potential capacity to love is just as great as those who actually had the child and lost it.

The grief experienced may be considered somewhat like that of the parent who has miscarried or had a child stillborn. The loss is very similar. It's the same as death, for their child will also not come to birth, and the parents experience grief. However, in a sense, it's an ongoing grief. Corresponding to that of the parent who has had a child kidnapped. Every time they see a child, they're reminded of their loss, and their grief continues so long as the kidnapped child is not returned. In much the same way their grief continues, as long as they do not have a child. Every time they see children playing, or pass a school, they're reminded of their own loss. Perhaps the ultimate form of pain for a childless mother is to have to attend a baby shower, or christening, and put forth a facade of joy, while she is dying internally.

Friends are often well-intentioned, but unthinking and insensitive to the pain of the childless couple. People who tell you to "just relax," and "stop trying so hard," or people that tell you as a doctor told us, "Just have a drink before you go to bed to relax you."

People, whom you meet socially often open a conversation by asking, "How many children do you have?" It's not uncommon for the pain and misery experienced to cause the couple to withdraw and isolate themselves which further compounds the problem.

My wife and I are painfully aware of the reality of the

pains and the hurts involved with the problem of infertility. It took about three years after we began attempting to have a child, before she was actually able to conceive. We too, for a season, experienced the *pain of childlessness.*

By way of introduction, I've asked Sue to share with you briefly our personal experience with childlessness...

SUE'S ACCOUNT

Today I still can not smell a certain brand of dishwashing soap without feeling a residue of grief and disappointment originally experienced one night as I did dishes more than twenty-four years ago. Standing at the sink, at the end of a busy day, I would finally have time to think and to grieve over my childlessness. Bill and I had been married four years, and had been seriously trying to have a child for at least the two preceding years with no success. It seemed ironic to me that this now desperate person with an unquenchable yearning for a child, was the same woman who several years prior had a powerful *spirit of the fear of childbirth*, and had earnestly desired to never have to go through that experience. Perhaps it had been my mother's often repeated warning, when I would complain of some kind of malady, "Just wait until you go through childbirth," or, her stories of how quickly and painfully my brother and I had been born.

Perhaps the added exposure to ridiculous T.V. and movie accounts portraying women screaming while giving birth had increased my aversion to the whole process. I only knew that now I wanted a child so badly, that I would have gone through anything to have one.

I sometimes think that a firm resolve to face fear, no matter how great, in order to reach a desired goal, can of itself bring deliverance. By this time I had lost the fear of birth, and had acquired in its place the fear of being childlessness and all that fear represented to me: lack of fulfillment, ostracism from

10

life's experiences with my married friends, disappointment for my parents, failure to achieve part of my purpose in life, and of a love never fully able to be given.

There are many of seasons of the year which involve children; holidays, vacations, and family get-togethers. They all served as reminders of what I saw as failure on my part. I knew that parenting had to be one of the most meaningful challenges of life; one I feared I would never experience. To my way of thinking, so many *undeserving* people were having *unwanted* children, and childlessness seemed to me to be one of the most unfair cuts of all.

The childless couple truly wants a child with all their hearts. There was no real escape for me from the constant sorrow, resulting from attending baby showers, receiving birth announcements, and the joy of my friends and relatives all continually reminding me of my emptiness. Even the polite jesting question, 'When are you two going to have a baby?' seemed to me to be unfeeling even though it was, of course, uttered by those unaware of my own private grief.

Fighting back bitter tears, my mind went over and over the words I'd heard from each different doctor, all of which gave us little or no information. The most helpful doctor had at least educated Bill and me on optimum times for conception, but we were still facing six months of failure, even with his progressive fertility program. There had even been a mention of the possibility of artificial insemination which somehow I dreaded.

The only real hope had come to me in a most unexpected place, my church. Back then I was a nominal Christian and knew little of the power of Jesus and His Spirit. But there was one Sunday when the minister's sermon featured the story of Hannah from the first chapter of 1 Samuel. I found myself completely engrossed in the story, and totally a part of her experience of bitter weeping in verse 10. I became remarkably

11

stirred when she made her promise to God, that if she ever conceived, she would dedicate this child to God all the days of his life.

That day I prayed the same promise. At times of my greatest bitterness, the memory of that day would return to give me strange and unexpected comfort. Finally, I began to realize that my depression was going to destroy my life if I didn't make some changes in my attitude. We can allow disappointment to destroy us and bitterness to defile many around us, until we get so tired of being that way that we want to change. This desire to pull myself out of my sorrow and self-pity began stirring in me after the Christmas of 1965. I knew I had to change or I would self-destruct.

In January of 1966 I came to a firm resolve. I would forget about having my own children, and devote the rest of my life to those of other people. I was an elementary teacher, and could foresee putting all my energy and talent into contributing in positive ways towards the futures of countless pupils whom I would have in the years to come. I remember the night I made that decision. I remember also the freedom I felt as I saw myself walk away from the grief and frustration. I even felt a burst of enthusiasm and a sense of meaning, and a surrender to the will of God.

Nine months later, almost to the day of my decision to relinquish it all, I gave birth to a beautiful son, Kevin, and two years later to another who is now tall, handsome Steve. Over my desk is a plaque with the words of Hannah's promise, "For this child I prayed, and the Lord hath given me my petition which I asked of him. Therefore also, I have lent him to the Lord, as long as he liveth, he shall be lent to the Lord."

* * * * *

Beautifully enough, in her recounting of our experience, Sue has hit upon a number of problems commonly experienced by women in this type of situation.

Satan attempted to frustrate our attempts to have offspring even after they were conceived. Sue had to go to bed for between four and five months with each child, with her feet elevated, in order to prevent premature labor, premature delivery or miscarriage. Satan's campaign to deny us children did not end at birth. He would later fight with us for our children, even after their births occurred. But first we had more to learn...

* * * * *

Our first encounter with a supernatural source of infertility occurred late one evening in our own home...

STERILITY REVEALED AS A SPIRIT

Deliverance Overcomes Charity's Sterility

One night about 10:00 after a particularly tiring day, my wife and I were just preparing to turn out the lights when the phone rang. It was a good friend, a young Spirit-Baptized woman of about twenty-six, whom we hadn't seen for nearly a year since she and her husband had moved to an outlying community.

Her voice was trembling and I could tell that she'd been crying, as she said, "I have to see you right away! I know that I need deliverance! I'm desperate!"

Having in the past received similar nighttime calls from distraught people, I started probing to determine whether the situation was really as desperate as she thought. "What makes you think that you have a demon?" I asked.

She blurted out tearfully, "I hate to bother you so late at night, but I *know* that I have a *spirit of suicide* --- because I decided to kill myself this evening on the way home from choir practice by driving off the Second Street bridge; but God prevented me from killing myself."

She paused for a breath and I asked dubiously, "How did *God prevent you* from killing yourself?"

Matter-of-factly she replied, "He had a nine year old boy ask me for a ride home, and I just couldn't let him be hurt. No one had ever before asked me for a ride during ten years in the choir. I really need help!"

I invited her to come on over...realizing in my spirit that God had definitely arranged for her to be able to get ministry ... not only because He'd spared her life, but also because our evening was free. Even though we were already exhausted, I knew we had to help her if we could. His grace and strength had recharged us by the time she arrived.

As we began to minister to Charity[1], I quickly reviewed mentally all the details I could recall of her situation: she and her husband were active members of a large Methodist church, both sang in its choir; although she had received the Baptism in the Holy Spirit about two years previously and had entered into a deeper walk with the Lord, she had been out of fellowship with like-minded believers since moving; I was also aware that her husband had been having an affair with another woman, and had been hinting at the possibility of a divorce for quite awhile. One of their major problems had been their inability to have children. Although the picture was rather grim, none of these conditions was recent nor likely to have triggered this sudden suicidal response.

----

1. The names and identifying facts throughout this book have been changed to protect the privacy of the individuals. The cases are otherwise factual.

Charity interrupted my reflections, "I have no idea what set me off tonight, nor why I should suddenly become suicidal; but I definitely wanted to end it all, and would have, if Jimmie hadn't asked me for a ride. My marriage situation is deteriorating, but he still doesn't seem to be in any hurry to do anything. It's all just so.... empty."

After we had begun to pray with Charity, had asked the Lord to guide us and to reveal the source of her problem, she suddenly exclaimed, "I just saw something that I don't understand at all. I saw in my mind's eye a house that I lived in before I was age five." She went on embarrassedly, "I don't know how to talk about this because it's embarrassing and it involves my parents."

I reminded her that her life was more important than her pride, or even her parents' reputation. Her life was literally at stake.

Seemingly reassured, she continued, "My parents always had pornography lying around in that house, but after we moved into our new home, just before I turned five, I never saw it again. I guess they thought then I was too old to be allowed to see it." She explained.

Since the Lord had apparently brought this to her mind, I decided to pursue it and commanded the *spirit of pornography* to manifest itself and to come out of her. I was also led to do something I don't ever recall doing prior to that occasion, I also commanded every spirit related to pornography to come out as well. (I must admit that at that moment, I wasn't even sure that there was such a thing as a *spirit of pornography*, although it seemed logical that there could be.)

Eight spirits then named themselves and we commanded each out in turn: the first was *pornography*, the next *foolish-*

15

ness and then *harlotry*.[1] This dear, sweet girl was clean cut, soft spoken, gentle and refined. However, one thing that had always seemed out of place was her clothing. She always appeared to be dressed suggestively, in sweaters that were too small, or blouses cut too low, and skirts or slacks that were too tight.

I suddenly realized the obvious in light of what we were discovering in the spiritual realm, she had been dressing like a pin-up, or similar to the pornographic pictures which she'd seen in her childhood (and which she probably thought that her parents, or at least her father, admired). In previous ministry I had counseled with Charity concerning her "suggestive" clothing as being inappropriate for certain functions, and as being out of character with both her character and her witness. She had explained it away as being "the way her husband wanted her to dress," citing examples where he had even gone shopping with her and picked out some of her clothing. (Probably indicative of problems on his part.)

Each spirit was commanded to leave as soon as its presence (name) was revealed. I was dumbfounded when I addressed the seventh spirit, "you next spirit name yourself and come out of her," and heard it respond with a whine ... "I am the spirit of *STERILITY*." I was shocked because I had never dreamt that sterility could be a spirit, having always thought of it as a purely physical condition. The shock was also a pleasant one, in the sense that it could so logically explain why they had been incapable of having children.

Although at first I was somewhat concerned that some other spirit might be lying to us, I sternly commanded *sterility* to leave and it did. Then *suicide* named itself and was cast out.

----

1. I later found a Scriptural confirmation which could account for such a spirit, "Foolishness is bound in the heart of a child." (Pr. 22:15)

She began to laugh...she was free!

I told her as she left, that for me, the proof of deliverance is not a matter of whether or not the person coughed, gagged, belched, yawned or manifested some other symptom: the proof of deliverance is *whether or not the person can walk in freedom.* "The real proof of the validity of your deliverance from *sterility* will be when you have your first child. Please send me a picture when you have that first baby."

For me the fruit of deliverance is whether or not freedom from bondage occurs!

True to her word, Charity called me from the hospital the morning after her child was born to praise the Lord for His goodness and power, and to thank us for praying with her. She then sent a picture of a beautiful child. I have since received three more pictures from her, as God has abundantly confirmed the validity of His ministry to her.

On numerous occasions around the country while teaching or ministering in the area of healing, couples have come forward seeking prayer for the problem of childlessness. In those situations when I've been led to share Charity's story with them, most have responded that they identified with her situation. Many felt that it was a root in their own infertility situations. Most had themselves either been victims of, or had sinned with pornography, and requested prayer to break all ties with the sin of pornography, and to have the curse broken, and the corresponding spirit cast out.[1]

In the near future, I fear that there will be far more cases of sterility resulting from pornography, due to the influx of

----

1. For some additional possible spiritual causes of childlessness, see the book *Ministering To Abortion's Aftermath.*

17

pornography on television, and especially that which appears on cable television. Incidentally, we were never able to learn what triggered the spirit of suicide in Charity at church that evening. Something caused the spirit to surface. My theory is that she probably saw something that reminded her of the pornography. It wasn't a conscious recollection, but served to stir up the spirit within her. Perhaps something as unlikely as another lady in the choir sitting in a particular position or looking similar to someone whom she had seen in one of the pictures from her childhood. In any event, *"..we know that all things work together for good to them that love God, to them who are the called according to His purpose,"* and God wanted Charity free!

Four Revelations:

1. Sterility Was A Spirit In This Case.

2. The Spirit Of Pornography Was Received As Early As Age Five, or Earlier[1]

3. Pornography Was A Dangerous Door Opener

4. A Beautiful Spirit-Filled Young Woman Had Spirits Which Nearly Destroyed Her Life.

Most significantly from our current point of approach, the cause of childlessness in this situation was supernatural, not natural. Conception was being prevented not by a physical condition but rather by an evil spirit, or demon, that was both causing, and named, *"Sterility."*

Even before receiving this revelationary experience, we

----

1. For additional insights into the types of spirits and the ways they can enter children, see Vol. 3 in this series, *Deliverance For Children & Teens.*

had prayed with several couples who had been unable to conceive and had seen God grant them the desire of their hearts. So we had previously seen the problem respond to the spiritual force of prayer being brought to bear upon it, and had thus seen it to be, at least in those cases, spiritual in origin, or subject to being overridden by the supernatural power of God. Now we had been shown another facet of the problem which was definitely demonic in origin and therefore, clearly made within our power, as Believers, to intervene and over which to exercise control:

> "And these signs shall follow them that believe;
> In my name shall they cast out devils ... "
> (Mk. 16:17)

Although it was clear that we had authority, there were also certain natural, medical considerations....

PART TWO

"BE FRUITFUL AND MULTIPLY"

"Lo, children are an heritage of the Lord: and the fruit of the womb is his reward." (Psa. 127:3)

PART TWO

"BE FRUITFUL AND MULTIPLY"

THE GIFT OF REPRODUCTION

From the very beginning, we were told that we were created in the image and likeness of God. One of the earliest commandments that He gave us was to be fruitful and multiply. So clearly, reproduction is a part of that which God intended for His people.

Satan hates the gift of reproduction, which God has given to man. He hates it for several reasons. It is an act he cannot duplicate. He can only pervert, distort, and attempt to corrupt it in a desire to rob man of its blessings and benefits. In addition, each time Satan is able to frustrate conception, he eliminates a potential worker for the kingdom of God. Delaying, perhaps, the inevitable, and delaying the fulfillment and completion of that ultimate number of souls that shall be saved.

Although Satan isn't able to completely frustrate the reproductive process, he attempts to surround it with as much of a corruptive taint, perversion, and an aura of impurity as he can. Sexual sins, committed either before the act of marriage or after the act of marriage, tend to weaken the marriage union, cause doubts and fears, a lack of communication, a lack of intimacy, and otherwise impair the relationship.

Sexual sin, of course, also opens the individual to the possibility of the various venereal diseases, and sexually transmitted diseases. These can themselves function as a self-inflicted judgment upon the sin, further frustrating and impairing the individual's ability to conceive.

ARE CHILDREN FOR YOU

It is important to be sure that you really want a child. Both logic and honesty dictate that we consider one other possible factor that may affect child bearing. All couples who marry are not automatically candidates to be good parents, for at least three reasons:

1.) There are certain people who may not be particularly suited for parenthood. Both partners in the marriage may have fulfilling careers, and may be happier without the concerns necessitated by family responsibilities. They may have married later in life.

Some who are childless have shared with me that although others (relatives, friends, etc.) are continually promoting the issue, they themselves feel quite satisfied and fulfilled without children. So we need to be careful not to fall into the trap of assuming that every couple, or every woman must have a child to be fulfilled any more than it is necessary for every man or woman to marry to be normal. Some are happier in that state, and some may be called to it.

2.) Paul speaks of celibacy as a calling. Some individuals may be called of the Lord ("invited" might sound less compulsory) to a life of celibacy. Not in a perverted legalistic sense as we normally have seen it, but rather, in a sense of freeing from all responsibility in order to be able to pursue, unencumbered by family cares and responsibility, a rewarding career or service to our King.

3.) Not to be overlooked in our consideration also, is the sovereignty of God. God is sovereign, and may bless whom He chooses, and deny or likewise delay blessings for others. Many times the issue of infertility has not been successfully resolved by the affected individuals until they have chosen to surrender their own wills to the will of God. Having attained this latter submitted, or yielded state, the answer has often come with surprising ease and dispatch. It seems far easier, somehow, for God to bless the yielded, submitted vessel with uplifted cup (to receive the blessing) than one with an uplifted clenched fist.

One young man related to me recently an account of a blessed but painful experience that he had which he felt beneficially affected the course of his life. He had a vision while working away from home on a job that separated him from his fiancee. In his vision he clearly saw himself and his fiancee holding hands. They were gently joined by a beautiful little blond-haired girl, who appeared to be about three or four years old.

"I felt a love for that little girl, which remains to this day," he said, tears filling his eyes. "Then after a few moments she began to fade and vanished away. The understanding or interpretation that I was granted of this vision was, that if I were to marry my fiancee, we would have the blond-haired daughter, but that she would die while still a little girl. This vision was a definite factor in my breaking off the engagement. I later met and married a lovely woman and had three sons (no daughters)."

"My former fiancee, I later found out, did give birth to a blond-haired daughter. Oddly enough, I felt no compulsion having had the vision to obey its implied message to me. I was comfortably aware that I could still marry her or not. The Lord seemed to convey to me that the final choice was still mine in spite of His warning in the vision."

25

It is also interesting to note that he did not feel compelled to obey the implied warning of the vision. A scriptural example of a similar situation is to be found in the case of Paul whom in Acts was warned repeatedly of the dangers awaiting him in Jerusalem: yet Paul determined to go to Jerusalem, in spite of the danger and *in spite of the warnings*. God apparently allowed Paul the final decision as to his journey. (God by virtue of His foreknowledge, did know in advance the decision which Paul would make.)

Although the young man's interpretation of his dream or vision seems to go beyond the actual facts that we might observe in it, I believe his interpretation to be correct. The rather lengthy interpretation being somewhat parenthetic to the facts revealed, is perhaps similar to the way the Holy Spirit may give a three minute interpretation to a thirty second message in tongues. Some of the brief visions in scripture may take a chapter to explain, as for example, the finger writing on the wall or Daniel's vision of the statue of the man with feet of clay.

CHILDREN ARE INTENDED AS A BLESSING

Children are, and always have been considered to be a blessing, in almost every culture that has ever existed, and are especially considered to be such in the Scripture. God through His Word has indicated that He intended for our children to be a blessing for us in passages such as the following:

> "As arrows are in the hand of a mighty man; so
> are children of the youth. Happy is the man
> that hath his quiver full of them."
> (Psa. 127:4,5a)

> "Lo, children are an heritage of the Lord: and
> the fruit of the womb is his reward."
> (Psa. 127:3)

"Children's children are the crown of old men;
and the glory of children are their fathers."
(Prov. 17:6)

"And all thy children shall be taught of the
Lord; and great shall be the peace of thy children." (Isa. 54:13)

In the Old Testament we find godly husbands praying for
their wives to conceive and as a result:
Sarah was blessed. "And I will bless her and give thee
a son also," (Gen. 17:16).
Rebecca was similarly blessed. (Gen. 25:21)
Likewise Hannah was blessed. (1 Sam. 1:27)

Clearly, God intended the children to be a heritage in these
examples. In these instances and in thousands of other cases,
the children came as answers to prayer. God has, in essence,
defined children to be a heritage (blessing). However, we have
redefined that definition, since we no longer live in an agricul-
tural society, in which children are prized as an economic
asset, nor considered to be the blessing they once were.

Partly as a result of such thinking, family size has been
limited or restricted, through the use of a variety of means. A
recent study indicates that apparently new parents consider the
ideal family in America to now be one in which they have two
children, one of either sex. The study also indicated a confirming statistic that couples who have two offspring of the same
sex are far more likely to have another child. However, in
spite of current vogue, the truth of the matter, is that God
intended for His people to be fruitful and to multiply, and
similarly intended that their fruitfulness should be a source of
pleasure and joy for them. Modern mankind has chosen "to call
evil what God has called (and intended to be) good," and has
even gone so far as to destroy, via abortion, these blessings!

27

EVEN BIRDS DO IT....

This morning as I happened to glance out of the window of my second story study at home, I noticed two sparrows mating on a branch. This wasn't an unusual occurrence for it had been going on, even though unnoticed by me, since the days of Genesis:

> "And God created great whales, and every living creature that moveth, which the waters brought forth abundantly, after their kind, and every winged fowl after his kind: and God saw that it was good. And God blessed them, saying, Be fruitful, and multiply, and fill the waters in the seas, and let fowl multiply in the earth."
>
> (Gen. 1:21-22) [Emphasis mine]

I was surprised not by the activity in which they were engaged, but rather at myself for never even having thought about the realities of their reproducing. In light of what I had noticed, as I mused over my obtrusiveness, I was struck by the fact that God from the beginning intended for reproduction, even among the birds and other animals, to be a natural simple, on-going, uninhibited process. One could hardly think of a 'sterile' bird, or any other healthy animal as being unable to reproduce. It is such a natural process. Except of course when man has intentionally interfered, artificially, with the process as with 'neutered' domestic pets or animals raised for food, and unintentionally in the case of those species which have become 'endangered' because of chemical or fertilizer poisoning. Nonetheless, the fact remains clear, that in untainted or uncorrupted nature, God's plan for each species to reproduce 'after its kind' has continued instinctively, without effort or complications.

It seems mankind alone has managed to create complications within the reproductive process. Probably by some of the same means: artificially interfering with the process by introducing physical, or chemical problems and to these has added emotional blocks as well. The point is well worth noting: that God intended sexual relations as a gift for mankind, and intended reproduction to be a natural uninhibited, simple process (specific instructions were neither given nor apparently needed to accomplish the task).

MISCONCEPTIONS ABOUT CONCEPTION AND *MISSED*-CONCEPTION

When I was led to begin considering this subject several years ago for this book, I began saving facts about the issue whenever I came across them. I learned that there are a number of misunderstandings concerning infertility. One of the most common is that people think that when a couple is unable to conceive it's always the woman's problem. In actuality, in only about one third of the cases, does the problem lie with the woman; in roughly another third, the problem lies with the male. The remaining third is composed of cases wherein both the male and the female have some kind of problem.

Many people, including doctors, used to believe that infertility in women was 'all in their minds.' Today, nine out of ten cases are diagnosed as having physical causes. There is a brain hormone, prolactin, that can be elevated by stress, which interferes with ovulation, but it is rarely the primary cause of infertility. Most people believe that the infertility rate has remained fairly constant over the years. The fact of the matter is that twenty-five years ago only one in twelve couples were infertile. At the present, the rate is about one in five. The rate, having more than doubled, is probably due to the upsurge in sexual freedom, sexually transmitted disease, increased drug use (especially cocaine and marijuana), a general raising of the level of stress, and toxins in the environment, but the use of the pill, abortificant drugs and IUDs have all had their influence.

It used to be thought that if you were infertile, or had a problem with fertility, there was nothing that could be done. With recent medical advances, statistics show that eighty percent of males could be helped, and ninety-five percent of females. The point is apparently well taken, since at least fifty percent of those who seek treatment for their infertility will eventually conceive.

People also used to believe that a low sperm count indicated a lack of masculinity. The fact is, that there is no correlation between masculinity and desire for sex, production of sperm, or testosterone production. For fifty percent of men with low sperm counts, the suspected culprit, is lifestyle: overindulgence with alcohol, cigarettes, marijuana, sex or stress, all of which fortunately, can be altered. Although doctors recognize that abortion and sexually transmitted disease can cause infertility, in the vast majority of cases, they find that *the couple did nothing wrong to precipitate the problem.* Infertility is therefore clearly *not a punishment for some wrong committed.*

Another common myth is that the venereal disease, gonorrhea, is the most likely cause of infertility. The truth of the matter is, that the most prevalent is chlamydia, which has struck seventeen percent of the U.S. adult population. Regrettably, only three percent of those individuals who have been infected are even aware that they have the disease. Chlamydia can be readily detected and treated with tetracycline, but only if the doctor takes a culture to test for it. If the woman is not checked, and the condition is not discovered, it can destroy her fallopian tubes. Doctors in the field recommend that all women who are sexually active should be tested twice a year for chlamydia in addition to having regular pap smears.

A common misconception is that if an individual who had

30

produced children in a previous marriage, is in a subsequent marriage and there seems to be a problem of infertility, that the problem has to lie with the new mate. That need not be the case. If, for example, a marginally fertile individual had previously married a very fertile woman, and had a child; subsequently marrying a marginally fertile woman, the two, in combination, might be infertile. Normally a woman's sexual desire is greatest during the time of ovulation. That is the period when she's most likely to conceive, according to a study at the University of South Wales, Australia, by Dr. Harold Stanislaw.

The National Institute of Environmental Health Sciences has produced an interesting set of statistics which indicate that women drinking more than one cup of coffee a day, or the equivalent of other caffeine containing beverages, are only half as likely to become pregnant as women who did not similarly consume that quantity of caffeine.

Apparently there may be something to the old assumption that tight undershorts for men has an impact upon fertility. A recent study done at the University of Nebraska Medical Center shows that average sperm counts have dropped substantially since the 1950s when boxer shorts were replaced by the tighter fitting briefs.

According to statistics presented in the April 1989 issue of Dr. James Dobson's *Focus On The Family Magazine*, one couple in six discovers that fertility problems cause childbearing to be difficult for them. Couples are normally considered to be infertile when they've tried unsuccessfully without conception for one year or longer. (Webster defines "infertile" as "not fertile; not productive," and "sterile" as coming from a root meaning "barren," and thus, "incapable of producing others of its kind; barren.") Experts in the field hasten to differentiate between infertility and sterility, which is considered to be a permanent condition. The infertility statistics have ballooned in recent years because an increasing number of individuals are waiting to have children later in life. Many conditions causing infertility are normally considered by physicians to be hereditary in origin, and likely to worsen with age.

Venereal diseases, accidental injuries, birth defects, body chemistry problems, spiritual problems, fear of the birth being too difficult for the mother's health have all been cited as possible contributing factors to the current infertility situation by experts in the field. Even the seemingly innocent activity of jogging can cause a woman to become infertile, and can cause her menstrual cycle to cease, until she reduces or refrains from her jogging activity.

Upon considering these statistics, one is reminded of all the data bombarding us concerning cancer causing substances. If one were to believe all the frightening cancer information, one could hardly enjoy eating, drinking, or wearing anything or even breathing. Similarly, seeing all these negative sounding factors which may influence fertility, would probably cause one without a sound relationship with the Lord to despair, and to be left hopeless in regard to conceiving. Don't forget, our God is a miracle-working God! He is one who seems to excel in doing the difficult, and apparently loves to do the seemingly impossible. Remember also, that many of these factors which negatively influence fertility are *reversible,* if one refrains from the practice or activity (such as jogging) or the consumption of the substance (such as caffeine, nicotine). Recent research has indicated that even cocaine's notorious negative influence is reversible after three years of abstinence.

In several of the accounts recorded in this book, the doctors recommended that the child be aborted for the sake of the mother, or that the child, due to the health or physical condition of the mother would probably not be healthy, and should therefore be aborted. The mothers to be were thus advised by the doctor to have 'therapeutic abortions' based upon the results of prenatal sonograms or other tests. We have, however, heard numerous testimonies from women who elected to take the risk of undergoing childbirth against the advice of their doctors, and had beautiful, healthy children.

Miscarriages, stillbirths, premature babies, and the apparent inability to carry to full term are still far too common in our age of sophisticated care and medical treatment. We had a friend more than twenty-five years ago, who had twenty premature births. She only managed to have two children who survived, but they were healthy sons and today are healthy young men.

Treatment for infertility is often extremely expensive, and can run anywhere from two thousand, at the low end, to eight or ten thousand, or more, if surgery is required. Adoption is not an inexpensive solution either. Costs to a couple normally range from ten to as much as twenty thousand dollars before the child is legally theirs. The tangible cost is in addition to the pain of the wait, which commonly takes two years or more.

All of these situations and problems can function as blocks to the enjoyment of a normal healthy married sex life, and may impair the couples chances of conceiving. In addition to such relatively obvious and physical types of impairments, there also may be deep-seated sexual fears stemming from fear-inducing occurrences earlier in the lives of the individuals. Among such experiences might be incidents of rape, incest, or molestation which are far more commonly being encountered today as sources of sexual inhibitions than would be imagined. Along withsuch fears, there may be other emotional root problems. Some couples, and especially for those in whom no medical problems can be detected, may also be having children denied to them because of the work of evil spirits as we shall see in Part Three.

PART III

ROOTS OF DARKNESS:
UNDERLYING SPIRITUAL ROOTS &
DOORWAYS

"A curse causeless does not come."
(Prov. 26:2)

"Thus saith the LORD, Write ye this man *childless* ...
(Jer. 22:30a)

PART III

ROOTS OF DARKNESS:

UNDERLYING SPIRITUAL ROOTS & DOORWAYS

In the previous sections problems have been noted involving infertility, sterility, miscarriage, abortion, and stillbirths. We have come to discover that all of these can have spiritual roots and each can be the work of demons!

Why is it that some couples have difficulty conceiving while others seem to have children without any conscious effort? Are childless couples being punished for sins or failures in their past? Let it be clear at the outset, many who are childless are no more apt to be sinners, than are those who are gifted with children likely to be sinless. The answer certainly is no, and we would not wish to in any way add to the pain of the childless couple by even implying such to be the case. Our goal is certainly not to attempt to place blame, but rather to discover how to overcome any problems that do exist.

I have heard of cases of childless couples for whom, doctors, counselors and the couples themselves were unable to find any fault or other source of guilt. There are, no doubt, some cases of physical blocks to conception that may have resulted from birth defects, birth injuries or inheritance which obviously did not stem from any conscious wrong-doing on the couple's part. However, I suspect that if we were able to trace far enough back even in some of those cases we might uncover spiritual causes, perhaps in the preceding generation.

Especially do we endeavor to deal with those cases that may have spiritual roots. In the instances where sin has been a factor, it can readily be dealt with, forgiveness sought and received. God is able in spite of all the apparent impossibilities to heal any and all of these seemingly impossible and desperate conditions.

We have discovered in nearly twenty years of ministry, that there are, in some cases, inherited spiritual causes for sterility, and that there are certain sin related causes, in addition to purely physical conditions. A woman who inherits a *spirit of childlessness* is no more at fault for being childless than is the woman who lost her ovaries as a result of a surgical error.

So let it be clear that we are not attempting to fix blame, but rather desire to fix the problem. In some cases the repairing may require the ministry of prayer or deliverance, and in others dealing with a specific sin such as abortion. Just recently, a woman mentioned to me the case of a friend who had come to her in tears complaining that she was unable to have a child. The friend then said, "I told her that I couldn't have much sympathy for her, because she'd had three abortions a few years ago. Since she'd already killed three babies, it seemed like ironic justice that now she couldn't have a baby when she finally decided she wanted one."

I can understand the rather legalistic thinking of the friend, but her position is lacking in both love and compassion. Yes, the woman was certainly wrong to have had the abortions. They were sin, and as much as we'd like to believe that her sin was far more hideous than anything we've ever done, to God sin is sin. All sin is hideous to Him, but He is able and willing

38

to forgive any ("whosoever") that turn to him in repentance and ask for forgiveness. We have a tendency to want to see 'the pound of flesh' extracted for the sins of others, but want God to be long on mercy where we are concerned.

The pain of the childless woman who has repented for her three abortions is certainly no less than that of other childless women, and may be even greater. For she also bears the guilt and painful awareness that she has destroyed (killed) her three previous children. Put yourself in that hurting woman's shoes for a moment. Perhaps she didn't really realize what she was doing in the abortions, perhaps she was forced into them by a selfish mother, or by a jealous husband. We need to love sinners, as Jesus loved them, while still hating the sin.

God's laws don't always seem to work in accordance with our understanding of them, for God's grace is involved. Sometimes those whom we feel shouldn't be eligible for parenthood have children, and some who seem to be the most eligible, do not. There is a mysterious element involved, and we must recognize that God is sovereign.

Frequently, it seems that people in the world have less difficulty conceiving, than do the godly. It may be that Satan has no desire to frustrate birth for them because but for the work of grace, their offspring will remain in his 'camp' as children of darkness and disobedience. Since the children of the godly will enlarge the ranks of the army of God, Satan's logic and methodology are understandable.

Having ministered for nearly twenty years in the area of healing, I have discovered that in almost every case the physical problems have had spiritual roots. (*"The curse causeless shall not come."* Prov. 26:2b) The search to find the roots requires good detective work, much patience, perseverance, clear logic and spiritual discernment.

Thus far, we have already discovered the following basic truths: 1.) sterility and infertility in certain individuals have been overcome by prayer and 2.) Charity's problem was due to the activity of an *evil spirit of sterility*. Although we have repeatedly stated that not all problems will have a direct sin root, we do know both from Scripture (Jas. 5:15,16) and from personal experience that unconfessed sin can be a block to healing in some cases, and may need to be removed in the healing process. Therefore, let's consider possible sin-blocks of this type, beginning with the obvious.

A. SIN BLOCKS - Willful, as *perpetrator*

Many who sin seem to have no problem with childlessness. For those who are not sin-hardened, however, guilt frequently seems to be a block. It is certainly true that God can forgive any and all kinds of sins. Yet, it should be observed that sexual sins seem to be worse, and are far more damaging to the individual because they go right to the core of his being. From the moment of birth one of the first observations that is made about a child is either, "It's a boy," or, "It's a girl." From the beginning the issue of gender is a part of the child's very being.

Sexual sins seem to be more devastating to the personality, and have a greater effect upon the social development of a child than anything else. For some reason, the guilt associated with sexual sins seems to go deeper than other forms of sin. It is also more difficult even for deeply committed Christians to somehow accept the fact of forgiveness for this type of sin (or at least to experience the peace of it).

For some odd reason, it seems that even we, Christians, who should know better, find it far more difficult to believe that God can forgive our sexual sins, than He can any other kind of sin. It isn't logical, but it's an observable fact, as any counselor can tell you, that the deepest seated sins, and the sins which we seem to find to be the most difficult to accept forgiveness for, are those of a sexual nature. This is true even though we may know intellectually, conceptually, and Biblically, that they are forgiven.

I recently visited with a physician who made a very telling observation. He said, "Once a child loses his innocence, it can never be regained." He was speaking deep truth. Sexual sins tend to scar the emotions, and often have a physical effect. At the very least, the guilt associated with the sexual sins tends to knot up the individual's stomach, and can cause impotency, which gives another example of the kind of problems that can result. This perhaps clearly illustrates Satan's goal and methodology in attempting to 1.) prevent conception, 2.) prevent normal married life, 3.) cause hurt, 4.) frustrate normal sex within marriage and 5.) and to break up marriages.

In addition there are a variety of specific areas of sin which tend to function as sources of guilt blocks: fornication or premarital sexual activity, early childhood experiences of molestation or experimentation, contacts with homosexual activity, and the like.

1.) **Pornography** - Already considered in connection with Charity

2.) **Abortion** / **Murder** - Nowhere is Satan's hatred of children more evident than it is in the case of his attempts to murder children through the hideous forms of abortion which are being employed today. I will not mention the grotesque and hideous means employed to destroy the unwanted occupant of the womb. Any who are curious as to why physicians and staff are often reported to weep during abortions, might care to do a little research in this area.

We were delighted to discover that in many cases, when we ministered to women, and helped them receive deliverance from the spirits acquired in connection with their abortions, we were also removing a block to healing. Many who were previously unable to conceive, did so. Many who had previously been blocked from receiving other healings for themselves, were also healed.

Many women have been convicted by the truths contained in *Ministering To Abortion's Aftermath* and a number have contacted me to report having become convinced that although they hadn't directly had an abortion, they had *by the intent of their heart*, and in actual fact, literally caused the death of the occupant of their womb by the use of abortificant drugs, an IUD, or some similar means. Several women who have related having had this experience are now working in crisis pregnancy centers, and trying to help other young women avoid making the same mistake.

Many people living today have been born to parents, one or more of which have been involved with abortion. Thus, it seems appropriate to add a few thoughts for the one who has been born into a family in which abortions have occurred or been seriously contemplated by the parents. It is especially appropriate, since it's not uncommon for the offspring of such a family to have certain common problem patterns.

These may range from extreme feelings of rejection, to themselves later falling into the trap of attempting to resolve their own problems by means of abortion. In the former case, there may often be the corresponding attempts to get attention at any price, perfectionism, self-justification, self-condemnation, or hatred of their own offspring, all seemingly without any understanding as to why.

The appropriate corresponding spirits may also be invited in, when these emotions are allowed to flourish unchecked. Needless to say, such feelings or emotional reactions, not being understood by the ones experiencing them, will often be used by Satan to try to convince that person that he or she is mentally ill or a terrible sinner. The offspring who have themselves inherited a spirit of childlessness often feel as if they have become special objects of God's disfavor.

Many women who have had abortions in the past and some who have had only indirect contact with it, have subsequently found themselves unable to have children. Some of them have received ministry and been delivered of *spirits of childlessness, infertility, miscarriage, or sterility.* Numerous women have discovered that it wasn't necessary for them to actually commit an abortion: they became convicted on the basis of the intent of their hearts. The prospective father or mother who attempted unsuccessfully, or in some cases even seriously contemplated abortion, found that was sufficient to cause them to become eligible for the curse of childlessness. Note, pornography and abortion are not the only sins which can lead to sterility. There are numerous others as we will see.

Abortion is a Biblically stated sin apparently requiring a death penalty on at least two counts: 1.) as the "shedding of innocent blood," and 2.) as sacrificing one's own offspring. Psalm 106, in verses 37 and 38, covers both thoughts:

"Yea, they sacrificed their sons and their daughters unto devils,
And shed innocent blood, even the blood of their sons and of their daughters, whom they sacrificed unto the idols of Canaan: and the land was polluted with blood."

Additional roots of this variation of the problem may stem from some of the following types of contact with abortion:

Intentional, direct involvement with an abortion.
  a.) personally obtaining an abortion
  b.) paying for someone else's abortion
  c.) performing an abortion on someone else

43

Unintentional, indirect involvement with an abortion.
   a.) aiding, counseling, or assisting someone else in obtaining an abortion.
   b.) utilizing an abortificant, abortificant drugs, pills, etc. The intent of the heart, being to avoid pregnancy, even though the individual may perhaps be unaware of the destruction of the impregnated egg, or the abortion thereof, caused by the drug.

Forgiveness is available for all types of sin. It is available to those who repent of having had abortions, and to those who repent and seek it for the use of any abortificant means.

   3.) **Fornication** - Engaging in voluntary sexual relations without benefit of marriage, includes pre-marital sex.

   4.) **Adultery** - Engaging in voluntary sexual relations while one or both parties are married to someone else; even if "justifiable." One woman refused to confess her adulterous affair as sin, because it had "saved her marriage."

   5.) **Prostitution** - Engaging in promiscuous sexual intercourse without benefit of marriage, for compensation or pay.
   a. Harlotry - To behave like a prostitute.
   b. Seduction - To persuade or tempt someone else to disobedience, to do something illegal or immoral; to lead astray: to entice to sexual intercourse.

   6.) **Homosexuality/Lesbianism** - Individuals "leaving the natural use," burning "in their lust one toward another," and "receiving in themselves that recompense of their error which was meet." (Rom.1:22,26-7) These two "lifestyles" are themselves a judgment of God as indicated in the passages cited, but also may entail further "recompense," as well.

Sins of sexual perversion, or unnatural sex acts, can tend

to frustrate or by-pass marriage, family or birth. These serve as something of a substitute for a normal sex life in marriage. *Pornography* and *Masturbation* are two prime examples.

In extreme cases masturbation becomes an alternative for a normal sex life. We once ministered to a man who was so afflicted with this spirit that as soon as he received his pay check, he would immediately pay his rent so he'd "have a place to live" and would "put some money aside for food." Then he'd take the entire balance of his pay to an "adult" bookstore and spend it all on X-rated peep shows.

Homosexuality and *Lesbianism* are two more perversions of this type. These both tend to divert normal sexuality away from natural use, and usually circumvent the reproductive process, almost like a self-fulfilling curse. This is a great source of grievance to God, for it blocks his plan for mankind - to be fruitful and multiply, and perverts his creation.

Guilt resulting from prior involvement with any of these areas of sin can cause bodily reactions (p.e. muscle spasms), which may "pinch off" or close down part of the reproductive system. This occurs in much the same way that guilt or unforgiveness can produce ulcers.

7.) **Lust** - Internal compulsions causing guilt and torment, not necessarily fulfilled in outward actions.

8.) **Occult Involvement** - A major factor producing guilt in Christians, usually overlooked due to ignorance of the reality of the spiritual realm, is a prior involvement with the occult. There also may be specific areas of occultic contact which produce defilement of the individual or his home, as the following account illustrates.

Lois & Tom

Tom and Lois had been attempting to have a child unsuccessfully for about five years. Tom attended a seminar and heard teaching exposing the occult, and methods of occultic influence. At about the same time, he and his wife sought prayer for their condition. A scripture that rang true to his heart, was the one in which believers are warned to not even bring an accursed thing into their home, lest they come under the effects of that curse.

Tom suddenly realized that he might have such an occultic object in his home. His brother had been stationed in Korea, and had brought him a large statue, not made of jade, but of some similar semi-precious stone. His brother had told him the statue was extremely valuable. Tom became curious and went to several local libraries in an attempt to research the significance of the symbol of the statue, or idol, as he had come increasing to suspect it to be. He discovered that the statue was that of *Thalava*, an Asian god of fertility employed by couples who wished to have children. In accordance with the customs of their pagan religion, the couple would present offerings to the fertility god: flowers and food would be placed before the image.

When Tom became sufficiently convinced that his statue was indeed a fertility god, he determined that he and his wife wanted nothing to do with it. They decided to destroy it, even though that meant the possibility of not having a child by means of it's influence, and the loss of fifteen hundred dollars or more in value. So, he and his wife, in prayerful agreement, smashed the idol and threw the remains into the trash. He explained to me that he reasoned if he was to sell it, although financially advantageous for him, it might cause someone else to come under the idol's spell. Both his action and his thinking were in line with the Scripture,

"Neither shalt thou bring an abomination into thine house, *lest thou be a cursed thing like it*: but thou shalt utterly detest it, and thou shalt utterly abhor it; for *it is a cursed thing.*" (Deut. 7:26)

9.) Engaging in Ungodly, or Forbidden Practices

Disobeying God's commandments especially those concerning sexual relationships involving relatives (incestual relationships) can also make one eligible for the curse of childlessness. For example:

"And if a man shall lie with his uncle's wife, he hath uncovered his uncle's nakedness: they shall bear their sin; they *shall die childless.*" (Lev. 20:20)

"And if a man shall take his brother's wife, it is an unclean thing: he hath uncovered his brother's nakedness; they *shall be childless.*" (Lev. 20:21)

In addition to these Divinely arranged penalties, Leviticus 20 also enumerates other sins requiring the death penalty: sacrificing one's own offspring to idols (paralleling abortion in our day), sacrificing to or serving false gods, placing a curse on either parent, adultery, incest, sexual relations with close (non-blood) relatives, homosexual acts, having sex with an animal (bestiality), turning to wizards or seeking contact with familiar spirits, blaspheming the Name of the Lord, committing murder, or having sexual relationships with a menstruating woman. Since these are sins punishable by death, and represent an even more severe penalty, they still have the same net effect for the individual(s) involved: he or she *will no longer be able either to have, or to enjoy, children.*

47

God makes it absolutely clear that He desires to bless His people, but He also makes it plain, that if they refuse to accept and abide by His terms for blessings, that they will receive the opposite (i.e., will bring upon themselves the opposite of blessings) which are curses.

"I call heaven and earth to record this day against you, that I have set before you life and death, blessing and cursing: therefore choose life, that both thou and thy seed may live." (Deut. 30:19)

In this passage God is calling all the supernatural and natural forces in the universe to witness to the fact that He has offered *life* to mankind. He is also promising this offer of blessed life to the hearers and *to their seed* - to their children. God's blessings are "unto you, and to your children and...as many as the Lord our God shall call." This is also a conditional promise then, of life and health for our children.

10.) Sin of, Spirit of, Bestiality

Among the forbidden practices in Scripture which carry a death penalty, is bestiality, or having sexual relations with an animal. It is an offense to God for it frustrates and perverts the normal reproductive act, and He apparently did not wish it to be allowed to be perpetuated in the lineage.

Practicing bestiality usually either invites a demon or brings a curse upon the one who has practiced it. One of the common 'fruits' of this activity is to be seen in the offspring, who act wild and uncontrollable (described by parents as acting "like little animals").

Much of deliverance is basically detective work: there is a jigsaw puzzle nature to deliverance. Fifteen years ago I was confronted by a need for deliverance during a healing service and at the time was unable to identify the spirit by which I was confronted. However, as I set forth the truth above concerning bestiality, while writing this book, I suddenly realized the identity of the spirit at which I could then only wonder.

A woman brought her grandson for prayer to be "healed" in a service. She said, "He is retarded." However, he began to pace back and forth as soon as he was singled out. As he paced, his head made a pecking motion, and he repeatedly jerked his elbows backward, giving him the appearance of a chicken pecking for food. I recognized at the time that it was some form of a 'chicken' spirit that we were up against; that it was Satan causing him to manifest such animal-like behavior. But I had no discernment beyond that until just this moment, when I realized that a *spirit of bestiality* had entered and was the source of his manifestation.

THE SOLUTION

The solution for any sin of which you are guilty, is to repent, and confess the sin to the Lord, and to then ask for His forgiveness. It often helps to confess these sins in the presence of a trusted counselor, such as a minister or a very close friend. This seems to help break the shroud of darkness with which Satan has been able to maintain his hold over you.

"Lord Jesus, I confess that I have been guilty of _____. I am sorry for this sin of _____, and I ask you to forgive me for it, now in Jesus' Name. Amen"

B. **SIN BLOCKS - Involuntary,** as *victim*

    1.) Incest
    2.) Molestation
    3.) Victim of Sexual Experimentation
    4.) Seduction

5.) Rape
6.) Violent Perversion (ex. Homosexual Rape)

The problems associated with being sexually victimized lie not only in the existence of painful memories and subsequent fears, but also in the deep seated resentment and unforgiveness which pose serious blocks to receiving healing and deliverance. In the Lord's Prayer, we seek forgiveness for ourselves, and affirm our forgiveness of others before asking to be delivered from evil.

Forgiveness is not a feeling. It is a decision to release another from an obligation to you. This is a decision that we make with our minds and confess with our mouths, preferably in the presence of a witness. The feelings of freedom and love will come later, by God's grace, after we have decided to forgive.

One additional point worth noting ... *forgiveness is not trust.* For example, if a neighbor steals my lawnmower, I can forgive him for that action, but I may not trust him enough to leave my garage unlocked. You can validly forgive someone who has victimized you, without coming under any obligation to reopen a relationship of trust. Only God can show you when, or if, that person has truly had a change of heart, and deserves your friendship and trust.

The following prayer is for your use if you wish to forgive someone who has wronged you,

Lord Jesus,
I confess that I have harbored wrong feelings
in my heart against_____. I am sorry for
this unforgiveness and bitterness which I have
allowed to fester for so long. I now make the
decision with my mind, and confess it with my
mouth, to forgive _____, for wronging me

by _____. I forgive him to the best of my ability and I ask that You forgive him also. In Jesus' Name I pray. Amen. " [1]

C. DEMONIC ROOTS

1.) What Are Demons?

Demons are similar to curses in their ultimate effect upon an individual. Demons are disembodied spirits. They lust to have bodies through which to manifest their own lustful natures. The *demon of rejection* as an example, cannot be rejected until it is able to inhabit a human body which might feel or experience rejection. Often spirits work hand in hand with other spirits to accomplish their goals. The *rejection spirit* would often to work in conjunction with a *rejection-causing spirit*. The *spirit of rejection* lusts to be rejected, but that lust to be rejected cannot be fulfilled or satisfied until it is rejected. Therefore it's cohort spirit must do something to cause the individual within whom it dwells to be rejected.

As an example, let's assume that I am one with a *spirit of rejection*. I might look at you and notice that your hair is thinning. A *rejection causing spirit* might prompt me to say, "You should do something about your hair problem." or, "You must have some deficiency in your diet that is affecting your hair."

Whatever I actually said really wouldn't matter, and even if you didn't dignify my comment with a response, the *spirit of rejection* could still torment me with, "Did you see that look in

----

1. Additional teaching on the subject of forgiveness is to be found in Vol. 1 of this series, *Songs of Deliverance*.

51

those eyes? That blew it. You are just as big a jerk as I've been telling you that you are." The effect is that desired by these spirits working in tandem, to produce rejection, hurt, and torment.

Satan repeatedly takes something good and perverts it into something evil. He takes a healthy normal appetite for food and overindulgently distorts it into a spirit of gluttony. He works in the same fashion with sex, perverting what was intended by God as a "good and perfect gift" into something else. *Table 1* lists sexual sins or conditions, which may also be the names of evil spirits that have the same nature.

Sexual Conditions & Spirits

Adultery	Harlotry	Promiscuity
Addiction To Sex	Homosexuality	Prostitution
Amorality	Incest	Rape
Barrenness	Incubus	Seduction
Bestiality	Immorality	Sodomy
Cheating	Infertility	Stripping
Coarse Jesting	Lesbianism	Slut
Crudity	Lust	Sterility
Exhibitionism	Masturbation	Succubus
Exposure	Molestation	Suggestiveness
Fantasy Lust	Nudity	Unchaste
Filthiness	Passion	Unclean
Flirtation	Peeping Tom	Voyeurism
Fornication	Perversions	Whoredoms
Frigidity	Pornography	Whoremongering

Table 1

A Butch Spirit

There are a few additional related spirits that may be

52

involved in causing childlessness, which are more obscure and less obvious. The *Butch spirit* is one of these. Normally we think of a "Butch" (I really don't care for this terminology, but it seems to be the most descriptive) as the tough, dominant, or male-role counterpart in a lesbian liaison. However, the typical "Butch" type spirit can be observed in the case of the typical 'grown up,' or adult, tomboy. In college we jokingly referred to them as 'girl-' or 'lady-jocks.' The classic cases were usually readily recognizable by their well developed, muscular bodies, their involvement in athletic activities, close-cropped hair, and an aversion to feminine apparel.

A common case would be the individual raised in an environment that fostered confusion as to her gender. Typically, she was a girl born to parents, one or both of whom wanted a boy. As a result, the parents may have either consciously or subconsciously treated her, and perhaps even dressed her as a boy. In other cases, the girl was born as a second or third child in a family which doted upon, or idolized one of her older brothers. She continually heard, "Act like John," or, "You should be a good student, like John."

It became apparent to her that John could do no wrong, and that her parents preferred, or favored John. Thus, naturally enough the girl endeavored, again either consciously or subconsciously to emulate John: to literally "be like John." She chose to mimic him and may even have found herself dressing like him. She tries to act and look like John to obtain the attention and approval of her parents.

What began as simply "being a tomboy," later became a lifestyle, a habitual (albeit often subconsciously) dress pattern of not appearing feminine. The dress is really not important, except for the clue which it offers, which can indicate the presence of, or be symptomatic of, the presence of a *masculine spirit*. This will often be accompanied by a fear of lesbianism, or a fear of actually being the wrong sex. The enemy usually has planted the doubt that "There must be something wrong with you; you don't act like a girl; you're a boy trapped in a girl's body," or something of the sort.

An Effeminate Spirit

The corresponding type of spirit that would operate in a male under similar circumstances would be an *effeminate spirit*. I once visited with an Assembly of God minister who related to me an experience that occurred one evening as he was preaching during a revival. He noticed the twenty-six year old son of one of the elders who had just been forcibly brought home by his parents sitting at the aisle end of a pew. He said , "I knew in my spirit that the boy had a *transvestite spirit*. He would run off and later be found wearing lipstick and women's clothing."

Even though it didn't agree with his denomination's theology, he felt the Holy Spirit move upon him to cast out the spirit. He said, "I commanded that *transvestite spirit* to come out of the boy and it did! You could tell it because the boy gagged a few times, coughed, and then you could see the 'release' written all over his face. The next morning his father called to tell me that the boy had face hair (beard hair) appear overnight, that he had to shave for the first time in his life." [1]

I continue to be amazed at the physical effect spirits can have upon the human body. However, we should remember that if a spirit can retard the growth of facial hair on a young man, another spirit could certainly retard the growth of a fetus, prevent conception, or curtail fertility.

----

1. Another account of a *spirit of homosexuality* being cast out is recorded in Vol. 1 *Songs of Deliverance*.

54

2.) <u>What</u> <u>Are</u> <u>The</u> <u>Goals</u> <u>of</u> L

Demons have something far more in.
merely make one feel bad, although they sp.
time and effort in this category of activity. Th
plan assigned to them by their commander-in-ci.
apparently three-fold. Their first and primary goal is
a person from accepting Jesus as Lord and Savior. ı   .g to
accomplish the primary goal, then the secondary goal is to
prevent the believer from serving Jesus at all, if possible, or, at
the least, to minimize the person's effectiveness as a believer.
They attempt to prevent him serving up to his potential. Third-
ly, if the former goals have been unattainable, the demons
attempt to cause the believer to turn away from God, to deny
Jesus, to come to a point of serving Satan, or, if possible, to
destroy him or her. It is certainly unpleasant to think that we
have an enemy who is so ruthless and so dedicated to our
destruction, but we do!

We must not be ignorant of the wiles of the enemy.

A specific goal of demons, in the area of reproduction, is
to pervert the reproductive process, to cause perverse thoughts
and/or sin to corrupt the reproductive act, and to prevent or
frustrate normal healthy procreation. If Satan can prevent a
child being born that means one less potential believer with
which he has to deal, in addition to the torment and frustration
caused for the would be parents.

Jesus Himself makes it clear to us that demons can cause a
physical effect upon the human body. He does so in the thir-
teenth chapter of Luke, as He ministered to the crippled
woman; when He stated that "Satan had her bound," cast the
spirit of infirmity out, and at the same time "loosed" her from
her infirmity making her completely whole. Thus, it is a Biblical fact that an evil or unclean spirit can cause physical problems; that lying deep underneath a medically diagnosed physi-

...rder may be a spiritual root. Doctors can treat the ...tward symptoms, but the Holy Spirit through the Name of Jesus serves as a searchlight that brings deliverance from the deep underlying spirits of darkness. [1]

That demons can cause blindness is clear from the Scripture (Mt. 12:22). By way of confirmation, Gordon Lindsay, founder of Christ For The Nations in Dallas, once described a situation he had encountered in ministering to a man suffering from blindness. He said the Holy Spirit enabled him to discern a demon sitting on, and pinching off the optic nerve of the blind man. The spirit was cast out, and the man was able to see.

If a demon can cause blindness in that fashion, then a demon could certainly cause sterility by pinching off a tube in either the man or the woman. Naturally the medical profession, not recognizing the truths of which we speak, would attempt to treat the lack of sight problem surgically. Similarly, they do not recognize the possibility of a demonic root causing either infertility or sterility, thus can only recommend medical options, such as surgery, drugs or in vitro solutions.

3.) Specific Blocking Spirits

Any of the above areas of unconfessed sin can give entry to a spirit of the same name or related nature. Spirits are usually found in groups. They will often draw (or invite), when allowed to remain unchallenged, other similar or related spirits. As an example a *spirit of pornography* may draw in spirits of *lust, whoremongering, fornication, adultery, or sterility,* as we have seen. However, specifically there are four main types of spirit that negatively influence the ability to conceive and bear

----

1. For additional insights into the workings of deliverance, we suggest Vol. 1 in this series, *Songs Of Deliverance.*

children.

      a.) Frigidity
      b.) Infertility
      c.) Sterility
      d.) Miscarriage

Frigidity in the above list is used in a broad sense to cover a broad spectrum of other spirits which impart inhibitions impairing normal enjoyment of intercourse.

Demons can enter in childhood due to forces beyond a person's control, for example as a result of the sin of parents or grand-parents, or traumatic personal experiences.[1] Among such experiences might be incidents of rape, incest, or molestation which are far more commonly being encountered today as sources of sexual inhibitions than would be imagined. In addition to such fears, there may be other emotional root problems. Some couples may also be having children denied to them because of the work of evil spirits.

4.) Further Complications

a.) Complications of Bitterness

In the Scripture we find the account of Hannah who had to release *bitterness* (I Sam. 1:10 "wept bitterly"). Bitterness is deep resentment and anger stemming from the feeling of having been cheated; seeing yourself denied what others possess or have easily acquired. This is one of the reasons why adoption of one child can trigger the natural conception of another. Once the feeling of being cheated or denied has abated, deliverance

----

1. Extensive information on this type of entry may be found in Vol. 3 in this series, *Deliverance For Children & Teens*.

and healing can more readily come.

This principle may also have operated in the case of Rachael, although it was not the primary factor stated in the Scripture. Nevertheless, once her maid bore her a son, she had a release from some of the bitterness against Leah, and did herself conceive.

b.) Complications of Fear

The very real stresses caused to a woman as a result of being childless and the accompanying fears may themselves function to further complicate, or even, cause the condition. They may cause a "pinching off" or impairment of internal organs, thereby preventing conception. Conversely, these stresses are often relaxed and the fears of being permanently childless are alleviated, when adoption actually occurs, or the decision is made to do so. This may be the explanation for the common phenomenon of women who were previously diagnosed as being sterile, suddenly becoming pregnant when the pressure is off them to conceive.

There is a great deal of fear and desperation associated with the awareness that the "biological clock is ticking." The calendar is a constant reminder that every year that passes is increasing the odds against the likelihood of conception. However, there is hope even in the natural: the most recent statistics released, show that women in the 40-49 age category gave birth to 36,156 babies in 1987. The most prolific group within this category logically enough was the 40-44 year old women who accounted for 34,781 of the births.[1]

It is possible for any of the previously mentioned spirits to

----

1. June, 1990: National Center for Health Statistics.

be inherited or passed down through the family. Leviticus 17:11 tells us that the "life of the flesh is in the blood." Just as many physical conditions tend to be passed down, or to 'come down' through the genes, medically speaking, so too can demons be inherited or passed down. Conditions such as spontaneous abortion, miscarriage, bodily misformation (tilted uterus, pelvic structural problems, tendencies toward tubal pregnancies, etc.), normally considered to be purely physical can also be the result of corresponding spirits.

As adults, we can open ourselves to the influence of, and infection with evil spirits by allowing sin to take root. When a family has a history of breaking God's laws, the future offspring can come under a curse as we shall see.

> "But if ye will not hearken unto me, and will not do all these commandments; And if ye shall despise my statutes, or if your soul abhor my judgments, so that ye will not do all my commandments, but that ye break my covenant." (Lev. 26:14-15)

> "I will also send wild beasts among you, which shall *rob you of your children*, and destroy your cattle, and make you few in number; and your high ways shall be desolate." (Lev. 26:22)

> "For such as be blessed of him shall inherit the earth; and they that be cursed of him *shall be cut off.*" (Psa. 37:22)

HOW MAY WE DELIVER OURSELVES?

As we prepare ourselves to approach God for deliverance, there are several things we should keep in mind. First, God is concerned about you and the condition of your heart, and above all else He wants you to be free to be fully His. It is important to be *teachably open* and *honest* before Him; remember that He already knows all about your problems. *Humble yourself* before Him, *confess* and *repent* of all your sins, *renouncing both them and Satan*, and every claim that he might have upon you. If you haven't already done so, make a decision and pray to *forgive* anyone and everyone who may have wronged you in any way.[1]

Finally, make the decision to *pray* and *use the authority* that Jesus has already given unto you:

> "Behold, I give unto you power to tread on serpents and scorpions, and over all the power of the enemy: and nothing shall by any means hurt you." (Lk. 10:19)

> "And these signs shall follow them that believe; in my name they shall cast out devils..." (Mk. 16:17a)

God has invested you with unbelievable power and authority. Having complied with the previous steps, now use the authority given to you and invoke the Name of Jesus -- command each spirit to leave you right now in Jesus' Name!

Prayer To Cast Out Spirits

In the name of Jesus Christ, I take authority over the spirit(s) tormenting me. I bind you now, you spirit of _____, and I command you to leave me right now in Jesus' name!

----

1. More information concerning the steps to deliverance and forgiveness teaching will be found in the other volumes of this series.

D. CURSES AS ROOTS OF CHILDLESSNESS

"Death and life are in the power of the tongue." (Prov. 18:21a)

WHAT ARE CURSES?

A curse is a demonic force brought to bear upon a person or family by the words, will or actions of another individual being. Actions of others would include parents' involvement in occult activities. There are two main categories of curses:

Curses originating with God, or *righteous curses*, which can extend to the fourth or even to the tenth generation of the recipient's offspring; coming as the result of sins involving the breaking of a covenant or the breaching of its terms, for example occult involvement or illegitimate birth.

Curses originating with man, or *unrighteous curses*, which result from words spoken by one individual manifesting hatred or ill will toward another.

1.) **Righteous Curses Of Childlessness**

A relatively common problem among couples where one partner in the past has been involved with abortion, is that of the *curse of childlessness, miscarriage or sterility*, as was previously noted in *Ministering To Abortion's Aftermath*. These spirits could also be passed on to their offspring. Thus in some instances, the curse of sterility may be a result of the individual's own action (as it was in the case of Charity), while in others it could be the result of a familiar spirit or of a blood-line (inherited) curse.

I have encountered both kinds in ministry situations. Having been involved in Charismatic ministry for nearly twenty years, I have been blessed to be able to minister to several generations within the same family. I have even had the glorious privilege of ministering the baptism in the Holy Spirit to members of four generations of the same family.

I have also had the rare opportunity of ministering to three generations of spirit-filled believers in two different families, each of which were influenced by curses resulting from abortions. In both families, the grandmothers had undergone an abortion. This provided a unique vantage point for me in being able to minister to each of the children and grandchildren subsequently born under the influence of these curses.

One case was cited in *Ministering to Abortion's Aftermath,* illustrating how every female member of a family became the recipient of a spirit of abortion, as a result of the entry gained by a familiar spirit of abortion. In that case Inez reported an abnormally high incidence of cancer among the women in her family, plus more than two dozen cases of specific serious afflictions.

The other case I introduce here, for it proved extremely enlightening for me, as to the way curses can afflict a family, especially in regard to reproduction. In the case of the Rose family, there was admittedly another factor which may have had an influence, that was some minor occult involvement on the grandmother's part in the past. However, by the time of my first contact with the family, the grandmother was experiencing a hunger for the Lord. Later each of the female members of the family and the grandchildren, three boys and three girls, all accepted the Lord and were baptized in the Holy Spirit. One of the grandsons is now in full-time ministry.

The staggering thing about the outworking of the curse in this latter example, is the unbelievably high number of physical problems and afflictions suffered by the women of this family, primarily *associated with the reproductive organs.* There have been instances of prolonged and profuse hemorrhaging (for years at a time), extreme difficulty in childbearing, problems with infertility, repeated female surgeries, hysterectomies, fibroid tumors, cancer, toxic shock, endometriosis, hormone problems, birth defects, dozens of ovarian cysts, caesarean deliveries, and PMS experienced by virtually all of them. This list would be abnormal for a large family, but there are only three married women involved. However, even the grandchildren have had many of these same problems, and several of the young girls have been prescribed birth control pills, and other medication in an attempt to deal with the physical symptoms.

Aside from the multiplicity of physical afflictions, it is important to note that abortion is not the simple act that it appears to be: it can adversely influence future generations. It can give an opening to a curse, and can lead to full-scale war against the reproductive process as it did in the case of the Rose family.

Especially when there has been a sin root, a demon may have been allowed to enter, or a curse to come into effect. I may seem to be going out on a limb in presenting this theory, but it is quite possible that such individuals have brought upon themselves a *"righteous curse"* from the Lord. Let's examine the first example given us in the Scripture...

a.) Abimelech's Curse

The twentieth chapter of Genesis contains a Scriptural principle, and introduces an example of a curse for disobedience.

> "So Abraham prayed unto God: and God healed Abimelech, and his wife, and his maidservants; and they bare children. For *the Lord had fast closed up all the wombs* of the house of Abimelech, because of Sarah Abraham's wife." (Gen. 20:17-18)

We can see in this passage, a truth and a spiritual principle that God would not have us miss. A truth that has been reiterated and a principle that has been repeatedly confirmed as I have shared these truths across the country.

Because of sexual immorality, [Abimelech took Sarah into his harem with the obvious intention of having sexual relations with her. The sin in this case was *intended adultery* even though Abimelech wasn't aware of the offense, God revealing the danger to him in a dream.] a righteous curse (a curse from God for breaking, albeit potentially, one of His commandments) was incurred. The nature of the curse was *childlessness* (He caused a "closing up of the wombs") that was brought upon the entire household of Abimelech, from his wife to his maidservants. It's a blessing to note in the Genesis account, that God's overriding goal was *restoration to righteousness*. In this account can also be seen, that God's loving motivation was to preserve all the parties involved.

When the sin was recognized as sin (being exposed by God to Abimelech in the dream), repented of, and forgiveness, or restoration with God sought, then healing resulted. (The curse was lifted.)

Clearly in this case from Scripture - *childlessness* was *a curse* resulting from sin (a specific sin, of a man looking upon a woman with sexual desires, then lusting, desiring her as a sexual partner even though he did not have a proper basis for such a relationship with her, through marriage). The action of sin associated with pornography is essentially the same - looking with lustful desire upon a picture of a woman (usually scantily clad or unclad) with the goal of deriving sexual pleasure from the act of looking.

We have already noted that such a curse was brought upon the entire household of Abimelech because of his taking Sarah with the intention of having relations with her (even though she was spared by God, speaking to him in a dream). Healing did not come until the decision to repent of the behavior, which brought about the curse was made, and God's forgiveness sought. However, do not miss the crucial fact: that *healing did come!*

b.) Coniah Cursed With Childlessness

To give another scriptural basis for this righteous childless curse concept, Jeremiah speaks of "Coniah" (Jeconiah) who was to "be *written childless,*" a curse placed by God upon his lineage because of his sin.

God always makes it clear what He requires of the men to whom He entrusts authority. He did so for Coniah in Jeremiah 22:3,

> "Thus saith the LORD; Execute ye judgment
> and righteousness, and deliver the spoiled out
> of the hand of the oppressor: and do no wrong,
> do no violence to the stranger, the fatherless,
> nor the widow, neither shed innocent blood in
> this place."

He gives him an additional warning in Jeremiah 22:5,

> "But if ye will not hear these words, I swear by
> myself, saith the LORD, that this house shall
> become a desolation."

God also states that the people shall know *why* His judgment has fallen upon the king who becomes the object of His curse, in Jeremiah 22:9,

> "Then they shall answer, Because they have
> forsaken the covenant of the LORD their God,
> and worshiped other gods, and served them."

God further states the sins of both Coniah and the idolatry

of the people who have found illicit pleasure in him, and then declares the dire judgment to befall him: loss not only of his rights to the throne, but also all hope of offspring.

> "Is this man Coniah a despised broken idol? is he a vessel wherein is no pleasure? wherefore are they cast out, he and his seed, and are cast into a land which they know not?"

> "O earth, earth, earth, hear the word of the LORD."

> "Thus saith the LORD, Write ye this man *childless*, a man that shall not prosper in his days: for no man of his seed shall prosper, sitting upon the throne of David, and ruling any more in Judah." (Jer. 22:28-30)

Thus, Coniah is one individual in Scripture who is clearly stated to be the object of a righteous *curse of childlessness!*[1]

c.) **Michal Cursed Also**

It is clear that a righteous curse of childlessness is not limited merely to men, for we see it employed in the case of David's wife, Michal, daughter of Saul. As a result of her envy, hating her husband for his spirituality (the less spiritual always hates and seeks to persecute the more spiritual), and for mocking him to his face for his dancing before the Lord, she was rendered childless. The Scripture states the resulting condition simply as:

> "Therefore Michal the daughter of Saul *had no child* unto the day of her death." (2 Sam 6:23)

----

1. He also unknowingly forfeited the honor of being in the lineage and ancestry of the Messiah.

d.) David's Loss Of A Child

Another less obvious variation of the outworking of the curse of childlessness is to be seen in Scripture in the case of David, who arranged the death of Bathsheba's husband:

> "And when the mourning was past, David sent and fetched her to his house, and she became his wife, and bare him a son. But the thing that David had done *displeased the LORD.*" (2 Sam. 11:27)

> "Howbeit, because by this deed thou hast given great occasion to the enemies of the LORD to blaspheme, *the child* also that is born unto thee *shall surely die.*" (2 Sam. 12:14)

Even though David was not technically "childless," the net effect was similar, in that he and his wife suffered the pain and grief associated with the death of a child and did lose their first born son. David's sin was at least two-fold: he committed adultery and then sought to cover his own sin first by deceiving the husband, and then when that failed, he resorted to murder. We see in this outworking perhaps a certain ironic justice, a death paid for with a death. David through his sin exposed his household to a righteous curse, noted in 2 Samuel 12:10,

> "Now therefore the sword shall never depart from thine house; because thou hast despised me, and hast taken the wife of Uriah the Hittite to be thy wife."

God, thus states both the curse and the reason for the curse: David's sin of despising God, in despising His Word or commandments by committing adultery with Bathsheba, and by murdering Uriah.

Righteous curses have many similarities in their outworkings with demons of the same nature or type. Although Scripture doesn't make it completely clear, I suspect that when a righteous curse is invoked, God's justice allows an appropriate demon to torment the recipient in accordance with the terms of the curse. (See Deuteronomy Chapter 28.)

"A curse causeless does not come." (Prov.26:2) It (a righteous curse) apparently can only come when the individual has *chosen* to disobey one of God's stated commands. For example, refusing to forgive from the heart and being turned over to the "tormentors" as Jesus related in a parable in Matthew.[1]

Righteous curses provide penalties for disobeying God's various commandments to men. God doesn't desire to cause pain or problems for man, but Divine justice requires a penalty for disobedience.

2.) Unrighteous Curses

Unrighteous Curses are similar in their functioning, to righteous curses, but differ as to origin. They are inspired by Satan. They usually are spoken or invoked by an actual agent of his or by one unintentionally utilizing his power.

It would appear that the outworking, or enforcing of the terms at least of the unrighteous curse, is turned over to a demon possessing the same nature as the curse. Although it seems offensive to me theologically, God may also either lift the blessing ("remove the hedge") or turn the disobedient, covenant breakers, over to "the tormentors" as Jesus implies in Matthew as mentioned above.

----

1. Matthew 18:34-5

68

3.) Contamination Curses

"Neither shalt thou bring an abomination into thine house, lest thou be a cursed thing like it: but thou shalt utterly detest it, and thou shalt utterly abhor it; for it is a cursed thing." (Deut. 7:26)

The type of curse which God warns against in this passage appears to be a combination of a righteous and an unrighteous curse. He warns us not to bring an accursed thing into our homes lest we become accursed. Thus, the end result may be either contamination resulting simply from contact with Satan's object, or judgment because we have disobeyed God's warning. In any event the principle is clearly stated: do not bring into our homes, or associate closely with the things of Satan for they pose a hazard to our well-being and state of blessing from God. In much the same way as other contagion works, or as dead meat draws flies, so too, we are warned that the satanic object may bring its contagion upon us.

4.) Spoken, Self-fulfilling Curses & Fears

One may make oneself eligible for a curse by committing deeds as mentioned above to bring on an unrighteous curse. One may also bring on a curse by the words of one's own mouth, or by one's own beliefs or attitudes.

In certain cases, we have encountered people who have been cursed by ex-lovers or by others, with frigidity, impotence or childlessness. It is true that there are evil curses which produce fear and torment that may be spoken against an individual:

by an enemy: "You will never be able to have children."

by loved ones in anger, or in jest, "I hope you'll never have children of your own."

by a mother, "You will probably have trouble conceiving, just like I did."

by a doctor, "You will have difficulty conceiving if you are ever able to. And if you do, you'll have difficulty carrying the baby full term, because of your structure."

by self, (could be a paraphrase of any of these others, or something like,)
"I'll probably never get pregnant because I'm too thin, too fat, too old."
"I don't want to have babies for I'm afraid I'll be a poor mother." Or,
"I'm afraid I might abuse them, because I have a bad temper." (Or, a usually unspoken, unfaced, vague fear that "I might abuse them sexually.")

There is a solution for all of these. Jesus has paid the price for us to be freed of every curse, and He tells us through Timothy:

"For God hath not given us the spirit of fear;
but of power, and of love, and of a sound
mind." (2 Tim. 1:7)

If you have come under the influence of any of these spoken curses, you may simply and prayerfully break their hold over you.

Lord, Jesus,
I acknowledge that you have not given me a
spirit of fear, and that you do not want me
under bondage to any fear nor to any man.
Therefore, in your Name: I renounce every

70

curse that has been spoken against me. By a
decision of my will, I bless those who have
cursed me; I now publicly tell Satan and all his
forces that they have no power over me for I
am a subject of the Kingdom of God. God,
alone is my King and I owe allegiance to no
other. I have been washed in the Blood of The
Lamb, and Satan has no claim upon me. Amen.

Satan, of course, is the source of all these potential unrighteous curses and fears. Satan also often curses the attitudes
of an individual with fear: for example the fear of having
babies.

Attitudes that are amiss can function just like a self-fulfill-
ing curse.

I had a friend in college who felt and often stated, "All
newborn babies look like monkeys, and I never want to have
any." He later married a woman with several children, and
never did have to have any of his own. Our beliefs, feelings,
fears, and predilections can affect or shape our destiny, unless,
or until, we submit them to the Lord.

These few examples, from hundreds of similar types of
fears and revulsion-causing experiences, should help us in
understanding how a woman can be perfectly healthy and
normal otherwise but still be unable to engage in a satisfactory
sexual relationship. Until the Light of Jesus's healing power is
brought to bear upon this area of darkness and torment that
remains within her (often hidden from her own awareness), she
remains blocked.

It is important to note: *a particular experience will not*
always cause a spirit to enter. People differ. With two children
in the same family who have had essentially identical experiences, one may become fearful, and the other remain unaffect-

ed. Also remember, having a spirit doesn't mean one has necessarily committed the act associated with that spirit. One might, for example, have a *spirit of murder* without ever having murdered anyone. In the same way, one might have a *spirit of adultery* without ever having committed adultery. A woman who is still a virgin might have inherited a *spirit of miscarriage*. The spirit simply is present in latent form desiring, and waiting for, an opportunity to manifest it's nature.

In many countries which still practice superstitious forms of pagan religion, especially those which employ witchcraft, it is common to hear of curses being spoken to cause childlessness, barrenness, or death for all future children. It is terrifying for a woman to be told that a curse has been placed upon her that will cause her children to die, be born dead, or that she will be unable to conceive. It is especially frightening for them in countries such as Africa, because they know that the curses work. They have seen the results. The witch doctors do a lively business trying to dispel these curses, often without much success.

The good news for the African woman and others who have been tormented by such curses, is that our God is greater than all the power of all the witches and all their spells, charms or curses. Our God is God of all! Jesus who loved the little children, still loves little children and those who would be their mothers. He has made provision to break all the power of the curses aimed against motherhood.

If you know you have been cursed, or feel that a curse may have been levied against you, Jesus is your answer and your cure! You may simply pray a prayer such as the one that follows to break the curse(s) against you.

"Lord Jesus,
I come to you as my Lord, as my Savior, as my
God and I acknowledge that you died on the

*cross for me. I also am aware and confess that
you became cursed upon the cross in my behalf, that I might be freed of all curses; that
you broke the power of Satan and of every
curse that his followers might invoke. Right
now, in the Name of Jesus Christ, I renounce
and break every curse that has been spoken
against me, especially every curse against my
being able to conceive and bear healthy children. I now confess that Jesus Christ is greater
than Satan and all the powers of darkness, and
confess that I am free of every claim that Satan
has had against me. 'No weapon that is formed
against me shall prosper,' for I belong to Jesus
Christ. Thank you, Lord Jesus for setting me
free. Amen"*

5.) <u>Curses Caused By Vow-Snares</u>

Many women have picked up fears of the pains associated
with childbirth. The fear of being seen naked, or shame can
cause stress and function as a block to conception, as can the
fear of intercourse, or of sexual contact. The fear of man (or a
fear of woman on the part of a man) can prevent conception
even before the fact by preventing intercourse occurring in the
first place.

Some fears may result from unpleasant experiences or
memories from childhood. Women have related being afraid of
sexual relationships due to recollections of hearing their prostitute mothers moaning and groaning with their customers and
assuming that they were being hurt. Others have recalled either
seeing or overhearing their own parents engaging in intercourse with the same result. Still others have related being
offended by the unchaste behavior of their mothers (or fathers)
and determined (vowed) *to never do anything like that*!

"If a woman also vow a vow unto the LORD, and bind herself by a bond, being in her father's house in her youth;"

"And her father hear her vow, and her bond wherewith she hath bound her soul, and her father shall hold his peace at her: then all her vows shall stand, and every bond wherewith she hath bound her soul shall stand."

"But if her father disallow her in the day that he heareth; not any of her vows, or of her bonds wherewith she hath bound her soul, shall stand: and the LORD shall forgive her, because her father disallowed her." (Numbers 30:3-5)

"But if her husband disallowed her on the day that he heard it; then he shall make her vow which she vowed, and that which she uttered with her lips, wherewith she bound her soul, of none effect: and the LORD shall forgive her." (Num. 30:8)

The Old Testament passages above tell us that it is possible for an individual's soul to be bound by a vow, specifically in the instances given, the soul of a woman. (Although the same principle of a 'vow snare' would naturally also hold true for men.) "Praying amiss" is a New Testament phrase that could include this same problem. The woman (or young man) who has been frightened by the possibility of an untimely pregnancy, and may have prayed a prayer such as: "God, please never let me get pregnant, and I'll always be good." or, "If I'm not pregnant now, I promise I won't have sex again, until I'm married." can give Satan a point of entry, especially if the promises aren't kept. Such vows, or prayers of desperation, apparently give him a legal right to block conception, or to enforce the terms of the "vow." Thus, these vows can become self-fulfilling predictions or curses.

It is essential to note that the Scripture states that either the father or the husband, if she is married, has the power to release the young woman from her vow. Either authority figure can excuse her, disallowing her vow, or setting it aside, and the Lord will forgive her because of their actions. If you feel there is a chance that you may have been bound by such a vow, you may renounce it yourself, on the basis of Galatians 3:13, or you may prayerfully agree with your father or husband in renouncing it, on the basis of the passages from Numbers 30:5 or 8.

HOW DO WE REVOKE OR BREAK A CURSE?

Curses to which you may have either fallen heir as the result of actions of your predecessors, or brought upon yourself may both be revoked with equal ease using the same basic truths. As we have noted previously, the solution for all our spiritual problems is provided in the Scripture.

"He that committeth sin is of the devil; for the devil sinneth from the beginning. For this purpose the Son of God was manifested, that *he might destroy the works of the devil.*" (1 John 3:8b)

"Christ hath *redeemed us from the curse* of the law, being made a curse for us: for it is written, Cursed is every one that hangeth on a tree." (Gal. 3:13)

Jesus was sent to undo the works of the Devil, and one supreme aspect of His work was that He not only redeemed us from the hands of Satan, but He also redeemed us from the curse of the law. An exchange was wrought by Him for us: he became a curse (took upon Himself all the effects of the curse

75

due to us) in order that you and I might become eligible for all the blessings which He rightfully deserved.

First, we must understand the basic Scriptural truth concerning curses as related above, recognize our part in the curse, how it came into being if possible, and our role in the breaking of it. Then, the following steps will be helpful as guidelines in breaking any curse over us, and will also aid us in breaking them over our families:

    1.) State or reaffirm your faith in Jesus and His completed work, which is your only basis for freedom.

    2.) Confess, if known, the sin that allowed it to come.

    3.) Renounce all ties with Satan, his kingdom, the occult, or the curse itself.

    4.) Verbally, preferably in the presence of a witness, renounce the curse. See the prayer which follows.

    5.) Thank Him for what He has done for you. Thankfulness is an expression of faith. Grace is God's "Yes" to us: Faith is our "Yes" to God.

A Prayer to Renounce a Curse

"Lord Jesus:
(1) I reaffirm you as my Savior and King, and I thank you for shedding our blood for me, which cleanses me from all sin and allows me to become righteous in the sight of God. (2) I confess my sinning [with pornography] which made me eligible for this righteous curse. I repent of my sin, ask your forgiveness for it, and your help in refraining from any further contact with it. (3) By a decision of my will I break all ties with Satan, his kingdom, the occult, or any other route of access that I may have opened to him. (4) I acknowledge that you became a curse for me that I might be freed

76

*from all curses, and I now renounce and sever
all ties with the curse of [childlessness]. I break
its power over me, my family and my lineage,
in your name and the power of your completed
work upon the cross. (5) I thank you for having
made provision for me in advance and for
having broken this curse over me. In your
precious name I pray. Amen.* "

Having seen all of these curses, demons, and possible
sources of blocks to conception, we need to have our faith
increased....

PART IV

FAITH-BUILDING EXAMPLES

"Jesus said unto him, If thou canst believe,
all things are possible to him that believeth." (Mark 9:23)

"...and *nothing shall be impossible unto you.*" (Matthew 17:20)

"For with God nothing shall be impossible." (Luke 1:37)

PART IV

FAITH-BUILDING EXAMPLES

In the Scripture we find accounts of nine women who were barren or who otherwise should have been unable to bear: Sarah, Rebecca, Leah, Rachel, the wife of Manoah, Hannah, the Shunammite woman, Elizabeth, and then finally the woman through whom the ultimate miracle birth was accomplished, Mary, the mother of Jesus. All subsequently experienced supernatural conceptions. [Additionally, there were women in at least three families who were barren, either temporarily or permanently, as the result of curses: Abimilech's wife, Michal, and the wife of Coniah.]

One interesting common denominator in each of the nine cases was the fact that each of them doubted. Their humanity was displayed when they doubted as the promise was given. Some laughed, some were shocked, but they all doubted and couldn't comprehend how the promised miracle of birth could come to pass. The important lesson for us to observe, is that *God's power is greater than the doubt of man.* Man's doubt does not block God.[1]

----

1. Doubt differs from unbelief. Unbelief *chooses* not to believe. It was manifested toward Jesus in His own home town town of Nazareth where He "could there do no mighty work." Doubt is merely an expression of one's inability to comprehend how something impossible in the natural can be brought to pass.

81

By studying even very briefly these accounts we shall see certain keys to their success in overcoming barrenness, and can learn from their experience.

A. NINE EXAMPLES FROM SCRIPTURE

1. Truths From Sarah - *The Grace of God*
Genesis Chapters 15 - 21

The cure of the barrenness of Sarah was a result of the sovereign intervention and the action of God, 'doing beyond her ability to think or to ask.' I'm sure by the time of the promise, she had ceased to any longer even pray for a child. She couldn't have even conceived of conception being possible. It was totally out of the realm of her thought that a birth could occur, or that her dead body could conceive. Yet, in spite of her doubt, in spite of Sarah's firm conviction to the contrary, (She didn't merely doubt, she was firmly convinced that it couldn't happen.) God promised conception, spoke it into existence, and it came to pass. In spite of Sarah's doubts, in spite of her *firm conviction* that it couldn't happen, it happened!

It was medically, physically impossible for Abraham to father a child at his age, and it was impossible from Sarah's standpoint as well. She was no longer capable (in the natural) of bearing a child. She was "past age"; her menstrual cycle would have ceased years earlier.[1] It was so implausible that when she heard the promise of a child she laughed out loud.

However, God *promised* that Abraham would have a son. It was illogical, against all reason. Yet God had said it, therefore it was believable! But still Sarah wasn't convinced and her

---

1. See Gen. 18:11

faith faltered. She tried to take matters into her own hands, to help God out. She sent in her maid as a surrogate, to provide a younger womb that might be better able to fulfill the seemingly impossible promise - that her husband would father a son. The faith of both Abraham and Sarah faltered and their level of expectation dropped. Abraham did father a child by Hagar, but he was not the child of promise.

Ultimately in the fullness of time, Sarah did have the promised son, Isaac. God fulfilled His word, and gave even more than they had anticipated; a child, a son, and a son who would be in the lineage of the Messiah.

Sarah, in spite of her doubt, was supernaturally caused to be fruitful. Her bitter experience of having been barren into old age was turned, after God's hand was revealed in the overturning of it, into a source of great joy. The very name of Isaac means "Laughter." So, great joy was the end result of God's intervention of grace.

We cannot overlook the role of Abraham in the conception of Isaac. He did manifest great faith, as the Holy Spirit comments in the New Testament:

> "As it is written: I have made you a father of many nations. He is our father in the sight of God, in whom he believed - the God *who gives life to the dead and calls things that are not as though they were.*"
> "Against all hope, Abraham in hope believed and so became the father of many nations, just as it had been said to him, So shall your offspring be."
> "Without weakening in his faith, he faced the fact that his body was as good as dead - since he was about a hundred years old - and that Sarah's womb was also dead."

"Yet he did not waver through unbelief
regarding the promise of God, but was
strengthened in his faith and gave glory to
God, being fully persuaded that God had power
to do what he had promised."
(Rom. 4:17-21, NIV)

A key miracle element that was at work in this case was
the miraculous creative power of God which simply speaks
things into existence ... or "calls things that are not as though
they were."

2. Truths From Rebekah - *Prayer of a Husband*
Genesis Chapters 25 - 26

Genesis 25:20, "And Isaac was forty years old when he
took Rebekah to wife." Recall the beautiful story of how God
supernaturally provided this wife, Rebekah, for him as recorded in Genesis Chapter 24.

"And *Isaac entreated the Lord for his wife,
because she was barren; and the Lord was
entreated of him, and Rebekah his wife conceived.* And the children struggled together
within her; and she said, If it be so," [in other
words, "If I am pregnant, why do I have all of
this discomfort going on within me?"] "Why
am I thus? And she went to inquire of the
Lord."

That's wisdom. When something is happening, and we
don't understand it, the proper thing to do is to "go inquire of
the Lord," which is what she did. This was a commendable
action and seeking on her part.

"And the Lord said to her," [He answered her
question.] "Two nations are in thy womb, and

two manner of people shall be separated from thy bowels; and the one people shall be stronger than the other people; and the elder shall serve the younger. And when her days to be delivered were fulfilled, behold, there were twins in her womb. And the first came out red, all over like an hairy garment; and they called his name Esau. And after that came his brother out, and his hand took hold on Esau's heel; and his name was called Jacob. And Isaac was threescore years old (or sixty years old) when she bare them."

* * * * *

Throughout most of the Biblical period, to be barren was considered to be an especially pathetic condition. It was the end of the line, an end of the lineage. Since there would be no male heir, the family name and the heritage could not be passed on.

Verse 21, gives the key to the solution of the barrenness in this case, which was the "entreating of the Lord" by Isaac. Isaac earnestly sought the Lord on behalf of his wife. Isaac prayed to the Lord for his wife because she was barren, and the Lord was "entreated" of him. The Lord responded, hearkening to the plea of Isaac in behalf of his wife, and Rebekah conceived.

Isaac, as the husband and head of the household, prayed and birth resulted, when he was sixty years old. [25:26] We note that they were married when he was *forty* years old. [25:20] That means a period of twenty years elapsed during which time she was barren. (A long period of time for a desire to be denied.) She lived with the pain, the grief, and the shame of being barren for twenty years. It wasn't a brief trial for Rebekah, it was a twenty year period. That kind of time frame tests faith. It tests patience, as well as perseverance and trust. But, by the same token, the delay, before the answer arrived, caused the fulfillment to be all the sweeter because it had been long awaited.

Note also that Isaac was not sinlessly perfect. His prayer was heard even though he was not sinlessly perfect, nor was Rebekah. That's important to keep in mind, because it's faith-building for us to realize that those in the Scripture who had their prayers answered in dramatic ways were not sinless, super-saints. They were people just like us with human problems and failings.

The proof of his frailty is seen in Genesis 26:6, "Isaac dwelt in Gerar. And the men of the place asked him of his wife; and he said, She is my sister; for he feared to say, She is my wife; lest, said he, the men of the place should kill me for Rebekah; because she was fair to look upon. And it came to pass, when he had been there a long time, that Abimelech king of the Philistines looked out at a window, and saw, and, behold, Isaac was sporting with [or caressing] Rebekah his wife. And Abimelech called Isaac, and said, Behold, of a surety she is thy wife; and how saidst thou, She is my sister? And Isaac said unto him, Lest I die for her. And Abimelech said, What is this thou hast done unto us? one of the people might lightly have lien with thy wife, and thou would have brought guiltiness upon us."

Thus, Isaac was not sinlessly perfect; nor was he a tower of faith. He was still riddled with fear, in spite of the fact that he knew that 'God was for him.' He'd heard the testimonies of God's anointing and blessing upon his lineage, upon him, the story of his own supernatural birth, and the supernatural arranging of his parents meeting. The Lord had also appeared to him and confirmed the covenant promise of "seed," and multiplied offspring.

Isaac also knew that his father had made the identical

mistake (or lapse of faith) in the very same country with another king who even happened to have the same name. His father, Abraham, had told the same lie (that his wife was his sister) to another king Abimelech nearly a century before. So, not only did he make the mistake of letting fear rule him, but he also didn't learn from the example of his own father's mistake. He was doubly at fault, both for failing to heed the example, and for his own faith being weak. Isaac wasn't a tower of faith.

It blesses us to realize that he was weak and human. We are encouraged by the fact that in spite of his weakness, in spite of his failures, he was still blessed by the Lord; his prayer answered and Rebekah was favored with a son.

3. & 4. <u>Truths</u> <u>From</u> <u>Rachel</u> <u>&</u> <u>Leah</u> - *Only God*
Genesis Chapters 29 - 30

Genesis 27:42-43. We see the beginning of God's purposes and plans to get Jacob where he wants him, that he might provide him the right bride. Esau has announced that he is going to kill his brother for what he's done in stealing the birthright. "And these words of Esau her elder son were told to Rebekah; and she sent and called Jacob her younger son, and said unto him, Behold thy brother Esau, as touching thee, doth comfort himself, proposing to kill thee. Now therefore, my son, obey my voice; and arise, flee thou to Laban my brother over in Haran."
Genesis 28:1ff "And Isaac called Jacob and blessed him, and charged him, and said unto him. Thou shalt not take a wife of the daughters of Canaan. Arise, go to Padan-aram to the house of Bethuel thy mother's father; and take thee a wife from thence of the daughters of Laban thy mother's brother. And God Almighty bless thee, and make thee fruitful, and multiply thee, that thou mayest be a multitude of people."

Jacob was sent to his uncle, Laban, because God was arranging the details for him to acquire a bride. The obtaining of his wife, was not quite so miraculous as had been the supernatural providing of a bride for his father, Isaac. This was due, no doubt to Jacob's sin of deception. But, in spite of Jacob's dishonesty, God still provided, and worked out the details to get him the right bride. God has a plan and a purpose in all the things that He does, even in the delays and in the desperation allowed to develop in His people, that they might turn to Him and all the more *wholeheartedly* seek after Him.

Here again we see a reminder, or an encouragement to be fruitful. Jacob went in obedience to Padan-aram to find a bride, and found there not one but two. You might say he was doubly blessed.

Genesis 29:15-18. He's gotten to Laban in Haran, into Laban's house and worked with him for a month. "And Laban said unto Jacob, Because thou art my brother, shouldest thou therefore serve me for nothing? tell me, what shall thy wages be? And Laban had two daughters; the name of the elder was Leah, and the name of the younger was Rachel. Leah was tender eyed; but Rachel was beautiful and well favored."

Leah was weak-eyed. She was not desirable. She didn't have the sparkle in her eyes that Rachel had. "And Jacob loved Rachel; and said, I will serve thee seven years in order to obtain Rachel thy younger daughter."

The time of his service flew by, because he had the goal in view, and was motivated by love. [29:20] Even so, Laban dealt treacherously with Jabob. It is ironically just, that Jacob, the deceiver, was himself deceived by his father-in-law.

"And he went in also unto Rachel, and he loved also Rachel more than Leah, and served with him yet seven more years." [29:30]

The one wife is the wife that he desired from the beginning. The other he was tricked into marrying, but they're both his wives, and apparently both of his wives, in spite of the promised spoken blessings of his father, are barren. Jacob has not one, but *two* barren wives.

"And when the Lord saw that Leah was hated, he opened her womb; but Rachel was barren." [Verse 31] That doesn't tell us for sure how long Leah had been barren, but had she not been, there would have been no need for the Lord to *open* her womb. It may have been during the full additional seven years of service that she remained barren. It may not have been. It is, however, definitely stated that Rachel whom he most loved was barren.

Verse 32, "And Leah conceived, and bore a son, and she called his name Reuben; for she said, Surely the Lord hath looked upon *my affliction*; and now therefore my husband *will love me*." She apparently recognized her condition of barrenness as an affliction, and felt that now that she had delivered a son, her husband would love her. We can empathize with these heart-rending words spoken by Leah, recognizing that she was not the choice; realizing that she been given a husband on the basis of trickery. She knew Jacob had been tricked or trapped into marrying her. However, in spite of that, she feels now since she has a child, her husband will surely love her.

We observe that several barren wives in the Scripture referred to their condition of barrenness as being an "affliction," or as a "reproach." In the statements of these childless women, we see a revelation of the way things are even today. Jacob's wife, Leah, said, "Surely God hath looked upon my *affliction,* now therefore [that is, because of my conception], my husband will love me." (Gen. 29:32) Rachel, in Genesis 30:23, upon giving birth to Joseph exalts, "God hath taken away my reproach [disgrace, shame]." Many women today feel that their inability to conceive is indeed an affliction, and many feel that the inability to conceive is an impairment to their marriage, and a block to the love relationship within their marriage.

Verse 33, "And she conceived again, and bare a son; and said, Because the Lord hath heard that I was hated, he hath therefore given me this son also; and she called his name Simeon." Again she's trusting that she will not be hated, this time because she has not one son but two sons.

Verse 34, "And she conceived again, and bare a son; and said, Now this time will my husband *be joined unto me*, because I have born him three sons; therefore his name was called Levi. And she conceived again, and bare a son; and she said, Now will I praise the Lord; therefore she called his name Judah, which means praise, and she left bearing."

Leah is trusting that she is going to be loved, and not going to be hated; that her husband will be faithful to her, because she's born him one, two, three, and now a fourth son. And when the fourth child is born, her attitude becomes one of praise to the Lord rather than simply *hoping* that her husband will be kind to her.

Chapter 30:1ff "And when Rachel saw that she bare Jacob no children, Rachel envied her sister, and said unto Jacob, Give me children, or else I die. And Jacob's anger was kindled against Rachel; and he said, Am I in God's stead, who hath withheld from thee the fruit of thy womb? And she said, Behold my maid Bilhah, go in unto her; and she shall bear upon my knees, that I may also have children by her. And she gave him Bilhah her handmaid to wife; and Jacob went in unto her. And Bilhah conceived, and bare Jacob a son."

In this passage, Rachel upon seeing the joy of another's childbearing envied her, saying to her husband, "Give me children or else I die." Illustrating both the frustrations experienced and the desperation of the plight of a woman in such circumstances.

Emotional conflict often occurs within a marriage, in connection with the inability to conceive as it did in Genesis 30:2, where anger was kindled, and Jacob responded, "Am I in God's stead who has withheld from thee the fruit of the womb?" In the heat of Jacob's answer, he makes the very common and seemingly true observation that it is God who has denied or delayed conception.

We observe in the first verse that Rachel recognized her barrenness. We note also that she envied Leah. The Hebrew word used here for "envy," carries the thought of "having born all she could bear." She was at the end of her rope. She even despaired, it would appear, of life itself. She was either to the point of extreme despair, or perhaps even suicidal because she could not conceive.

In her desperation, Rachel then attempted a worldly solution. People often get frustrated and impatient with God. "God hasn't given me the answer that I want, so I'm going to go to the world to get a solution." She, in essence, substituted another womb, that of Bilhah her maid. Her method was very similar to what we today call surrogate motherhood, or employing a surrogate mother, but the results would prove to be hurtful for her.

Next Rachel tried another artificial means. Verse 14, "Reuben went in the days of wheat harvest, and he found mandrakes in the field, and he brought them unto his mother Leah. Then Rachel said to Leah, Give me, I pray thee, of thy son's mandrakes. And she said unto her, Is it a small matter that thou hast taken my husband? and wouldest thou take away my son's mandrakes also? And Rachel said, Therefore he shall lie with thee tonight for thy son's mandrakes."

Rachel agreed with Leah to let Jacob lie with her that night in return for the mandrakes. Verse 16, "And Jacob came out of the field in the evening, and Leah went out to meet him, and said, Thou must come in unto me; for surely I have hired thee with my son's mandrakes. And he lay with her that night. And God hearkened unto Leah, and she conceived, and bore Jacob a fifth son." *God hearkened unto Leah.* This time we find that Leah's own prayer was heard by God. She was still praying for additional offspring; still trying, it seems, to woo and win her husband's love.

The mandrakes were one more attempt on Rachel's part to find an artificial stimulant to fertility. She tried the use of mandrakes, or as they are commonly called, "love apples." They were a plumb-like fruit that was supposed to have powers as a love charm. In a superstitious way the people of the middle east believed eating them would cause fertility. It was Rachel's worldly means to accomplish an end. However, as someone once said, "The situation was really in God's hands, and He could not honor a human attempt to change it." At the very least, God had a perfect time, and a perfect plan for each of the births of Jacob's twelve sons to occur.

Finally, from Rachel's standpoint, her prayer was heard in verse 22. "And God remembered Rachel." [*God doesn't forget anything, or anybody: every need, and every prayer is heard*] "And God hearkened to her, and *opened her womb.* And she conceived and bore a son; and said, God hath taken away my reproach." God heard the cry of Rachel's heart. He heard her prayer. He opened her womb, she conceived, and bore a son causing her to exclaim as had Leah earlier, "God has taken away *my reproach.*"

Based upon all the children that were born since her statement in 30:1, that she was ready to die out of her frustration and grief, it would have been a minimum of twelve years. The twelve years it would have taken for all the other children to have been born to Leah and the maids, would have been a time of great torment for her, living in a state of barrenness. Bearing still, the pain, the shame, the grief, the anguish of being without a child, while her competitor kept on having sons. Both women ultimately had to recognize that *only God* could solve their problem.

Many have similarly borne the pain and the grief of being childless for a season. But there are very few who have borne that pain for twenty years, or twelve years, as did Sarah and Rachel. However, we don't want to focus on the negative. We want to focus on the positive, and we want to recognize that the end result was fruitfulness. The end result was that the prayers were answered. Rachel did conceive and bare a son. God had something good in store for her all the while, but she didn't know it. We know that she didn't know it because she was in such anguish, that she was despairing of life itself.

God had something special; something more than she had asked for in store for her. He had something worth waiting for, even though she didn't know it. He had prepared for her a son, who would be a national hero, revered, a ruler of a great nation, and who would save his people. Her son would be a household word for his wisdom, even to this very day, more than thirty-eight hundred years later.

5. Truths From Wife of Manoah - *Divine Intervention*
Judges Chapter 13

The birth of Sampson is an account of pure grace very much like the birth of Isaac. His parents-to-be were also beyond the point of expecting or seeking a child. They were surprised by the appearance of a heavenly being who arrived with a promise for them.

The angelic being first appeared to Manoah's wife while she was alone, in an occurrence foreshadowing a new testament appearance to another maiden of Israel named Mary. Like Mary, she too, along with her husband, was yielded and willing obedient to the instructions of the heavenly visitor. Both the potential parents of Sampson were eager to receive the prenatal instructions concerning food and drink for the child.

We are not given the name of Manoah's wife. She thus stands for *any barren woman in any age*, who may similarly be surprised by the grace of God with a promise of healing for that condition.

We learn that Manoah entreated the Lord and that the Lord heard his prayer, but the prayer wasn't offered until after the angel had already appeared and announced the forthcoming birth of his son. So, his prayer, although beneficial, was not a crucial factor in obtaining the promise.

The angelic visitor did wondrously, it would appear that he supernaturally caused the sacrifice which had been placed on a rock, rather than upon a wooden altar, to be consumed by fire. He then mingled himself with the flames of the sacrifice, ascending with the smoke heavenward.

The heavenly visitor when asked for his name responded why do you ask it seeing it is secret? The literal meaning is "wonderful." Jesus is the One whose name is "Wonderful" and "Counselor" as we are told by Isaiah. This gives added significance to the visitation granted to the unnamed woman. I believe that Jesus is Himself concerned with everything that affects you: when you are hurting, He feels what you feel. He is concerned and involved in your plight. He is involved with your prayers and with providing the solution. Part of this is beautifully symbolized for us by His commingling himself with the flame and smoke. He identifies Himself with the sacrifice (He is the only acceptable sacrifice to the Father). It also illustrates His role as our Intercessor, and shows that He must be at the core of our prayers or of any seeking of God. It is only by, and through, Him that we may approach the Father.

Manoah is struck with fear upon realizing how great the Person was who had visited them. The simple logic of his wife should also encourage faith for others needing a miracle. If the Lord wanted to kill us, He certainly could have, very easily. He hasn't, and has instead, encouraged us to hope ... therefore, we should *expect the best*.

6. <u>Truths</u> <u>From</u> <u>Hannah</u> - *An Adversary Exists*
I Samuel Chapter 1

1 Samuel 1:1-8, "Now, there was a certain man of Ramathaim-zophim, of mount Ephraim, and his name was Elkanah, the son of Jeroham, the son of Elihu, the son of Tohu, the son of Zuph, an Ephrathite. And he had two wives; the name of the one was Hannah." (Hannah means grace) "And the name of the other Peninnah: and Peninnah had children, but Hannah had no children. And this man went up out of his city yearly to worship and to sacrifice unto the Lord of hosts in Shiloh."

"And when the time was that Elkanah offered, he gave to Peninnah his wife, and to all her sons and her daughters, portions; but unto Hannah he gave a worthy portion; for he loved Hannah; but the Lord had shut up her womb. And her adversary also provoked her sore, for to make her fret, because the Lord had shut up her womb. And as he did so year by year, when she went up to the house of the Lord, so she provoked her; therefore she wept, and did not eat. Then said Elkanah her husband to her, Hannah, why weepest thou? and why eatest thou not? and why is thy heart grieved? am not I better unto thee than ten sons?"

We note that Elkanah was a Godly man, who made the annual pilgrimage to Jerusalem to worship. One of his wives whom he loved greatly was barren. That he was sympathetic

95

and sensitive to her situation, and recognized the source of her grief, is clear from his question in verse 8, "Am I not better for you than ten sons?"

It is also clear from the account that Hannah had a problem with bitterness. The reason for her bitterness was that the other wife had children and she did not, and she was unable to because she was barren. The unfairness of the situation, caused her to experience bitterness as it has many others.

However, there is another important element in this situation that is all too often overlooked. It is the presence and work of Satan. In 1 Samuel 1:6, the word of God speaks of the work of Hannah's *adversary* in tormenting her because of her infertility. Most commentators have taken this to be the other wife, Peninnah. But in verse 7 the adversary is identified with the male pronoun, "he." The "he" to which the Scripture refers, is, I am convinced, Satan, whose will, and work is so often to be seen in cases of infertility and sterility.

I recognize that not everyone will agree with my interpretation of this verse. I can't even find a commentator who really had much to say about it. I'll just have to let the Lord make this relevant and confirm it if indeed I am correct.

"And her adversary..." I think her adversary is the same adversary that opposes you and me. The same one that would torment us, if we had an affliction such as Hannah's with her barrenness. There is one who is continually suggesting to you that you've got a problem; Constantly jabbing you, tormenting you, and reminding you of the nature of your problem.

The purpose of her adversary was to make her fret, to cause Hannah to worry about her problem. We have an enemy who is always there wanting to make us worry about our problems, whatever they may be; his goal is to cause you to fret. He can't fret for you, but he can cause you to fret, to worry, to get under stress and become anxious. "And he caused her to fret *because the Lord had shut up her womb.*" Whether the Lord had actually shut up her womb, or whether that was the only concept she could grasp, or whether that was merely what the adversary was seeking to convince her, the net effect was the same. The fact was that her womb was closed. She was barren.

There is no indication of a curse here, as there was back in Genesis 20, when the household of Abimelech, came under a curse as the result of sexual sin, which resulted in God closing the wombs of all in his household. That was definitely a curse allowed by God. Here it may just be that the enemy was attempting to convince her that it was the Lord that had prevented her from being able to conceive.

It's interesting, to note the change in gender: "And *he* did so year by year, as she went to the house of the Lord." Then it says, "So *she* provoked her." There is a change there, which may mean that the enemy had caused Hannah to start provoking herself, or may be implying that Peninnah was joining her real adversary in provoking her. It is probably more a matter of her adversary, or the evil spirit working with her adversary, causing Hannah torment.

Hannah was sufficiently provoked that she wept and did not eat. Sometimes when you're under a great deal of torment, food loses its appeal. Your appetite often disappears when you're under a great deal of pressure, or torment.

Although we can understand Elkanah's motivation and his rationale. In verse 8 we see an indication that he is unable to fully grasp the depth of the grief that she's experiencing because of her barrenness, when he attempts to comfort her with his question. We can also understand, that to her, in the bitterness of her soul, this was not real comfort. She couldn't eat, because she was in bitterness of soul.

"Now Eli the priest sat upon a seat by a post of the temple of the Lord. And she was in bitterness of soul, and prayed unto the Lord, and wept sore. And she vowed a vow, and said, Oh Lord of hosts, if thou wilt indeed look on the affliction of thine handmaid, and remember me and not forget thine handmaid, but will give unto thine handmaid a man child, then I will give him unto the Lord all the days of his life, and there shall no razor come upon his head."

She was in bitterness of soul; her soul was bitter. She speaks of her condition as an affliction, the exact same word that Leah, the wife of Jacob, used to describe her condition. Here we see the same word being used by Hannah to describe her condition of childlessness. We note that she vows a vow that her son will - if indeed God grants her request, and gives her a son - be a Nazarite from his birth. There are just three Nazarites-from-birth recorded in Scripture. To be a Nazarite was normally a temporary vow that a Jew took, but three individuals are stated to be Nazarites for their entire lifetime. The three were Sampson, Samuel and John the Baptist.

"And it came to pass, as she continued praying before the Lord that Eli marked her mouth." He noted something strange about her. She was praying silently. "Now Hannah, she spake in her heart, only her lips moved, but her voice was not heard, therefore Eli thought she had been drunken. And Eli said unto her, How long wilt thou be drunken? put away thy wine from thee. And Hannah answered and said, No, my lord, I am a woman of a sorrowful spirit."

"I'm a woman of a sorrowful spirit." She recognized her condition and the bitterness of her soul. When Eli mistook her praying silently for drunkenness, she explained it in this way: "I have drunk neither wine nor strong drink, but I have poured out my soul before the Lord ... For out of the abundance of my complaint and grief have I spoken hitherto. Then Eli answered and said, Go in peace, and the God of Israel grant thee thy petition that thou hast asked of him. And she said, Let thine handmaid find grace in thy sight."

Eli doesn't even ask her what it is that she needs, he simply says, in essence, "Let God give you what you have asked of Him." It would appear that she believed what Eli said as being from the Lord. There seems to have been faith at work, for she regained her appetite, and was no longer sad. So apparently she believed him when he said, "God grant you your request."

In verse 19 we note that they were a Godly couple. They got up and worshiped the Lord before they traveled. They then returned to their home. Subsequent to returning home, "Elkanah knew Hannah his wife, and the Lord remembered her." She conceived a man child, a son, and she named him Samuel. "Samuel" means, "Asked of God."

The balance of the story is well known. The following year Hannah did not go with her husband to worship saying, "I will not go up until the child be weaned." The Jews in that day normally did not wean their children until they were three. She would have waited probably three years before she went up to turn him over to Eli. "And then will I bring him, that he may appear before the Lord, and there abide forever."

That's really a tremendous action of faith on her part: to give up the child for which she'd prayed, unto the Lord forever. She would have realized that she would probably only be able to see him one time a year, when they went up to make their sacrifice. She was grateful that God had granted her victory over her adversary, and over her bitterness. The key here is that Hannah relinquished her child to God; offering Samuel up as a thank offering. She wanted her child to glorify God.

7. <u>Truths</u> <u>From</u> <u>The</u> <u>Shunnamite</u> <u>Woman</u> - *Ministry of A Holy Man*
II Kings Chapter 4:8-37

This account of another conception is similar, and yet in certain ways different from the others. The fourth chapter records the miracle of the widow's oil. Then a different woman is introduced. "And it fell on a day that Elisha passed to Shunem, where was a great woman; and she constrained him to eat bread. And so it was that as often as he passed by, he turned in thither to eat bread."

The Bible says she was a "great" woman. In what way was she great? She was great presumably in the sense of having position. She was a woman of rank, and a woman of wealth.

"And she said unto her husband, Behold now, I perceive that this is an holy man of God, which passes by us continually. Let us make a little chamber, I pray thee, on the wall, and let us set for him there a bed, and a table, and a stool, and a candlestick; and it shall be when he comes to us, that he shall turn in thither."

She had built for him a little place up on the wall of the house, where he could stay. She recognized that Elisha was really a man of God. He wasn't a phony, wasn't just out for what he could get. He was real; a man of God.

"And it fell on a day, that he came thither, and he turned into the chamber, and he lay there. And he said to Gehazi his servant, Call this Shunammite. And when he had called to her, she stood before him. And he said unto him," [Elisha, said unto Gehazi, not addressing the woman before him directly, but through his servant] "Say now unto her, Behold thou hast been careful for us with all this care; what is to be done for thee? Would you be spoken for to the king, or to the captain of the host? And she answered and said, I dwell among mine own people. "

In other words, Elisha says, "You have done all these good deeds for us, what can we do in return for you?" Since he was in a position of influence with the officials of her nation, he offered to intercede in her behalf. She, however, by her reply indicated, "I'm happy, I have no problems. There's nothing that I really need." She then left his presence.

So, Elisha inquires of Gehazi, "And he said, What then is to be done for her? And Gehazi answered, Verily she has no child, and her husband is old."

In his brief response, Gehazi informs us that she too is barren, and states a major factor in her barrenness to be the fact that her husband is beyond the age of being able to produce a child. A situation somewhat similar to that noted with Abraham and Sarah. The Shunammite is barren without a child, and the current status is, that her husband is too old to be able to provide her one.

Elisha sends Gehazi for the woman, and Gehazi went and summoned her. "And when he had called her, she stood in the door. [She returned to the doorway of the room] And he said, About this season, according to the time of life, thou shalt embrace a son. And she said, Nay, my lord, thou man of God, do not lie unto thine handmaid."
The Shunammite couldn't believe what he was offering her to be true and so she said in essence, "Please do not joke with me; don't tease me about this for I have been deeply hurting because of my childless for many years."

Once again in spite of the doubt on the part on the recipient of the promise, the woman conceived and did bear a son at the very time that Elisha had prophesied or promised that she would. Later this same miraculously provided child would die, but in response to her faith in, and relying upon, the ministry of 'the holy man of God,' he was restored to life.

8. Truths From Elisabeth - *Righteous, But Barren*
Luke Chapter 1

This beautiful account is perhaps one of the most significant and meaningful of all the Biblical narrations involving barrenness. It clarifies a number of issues and answers several questions.

One of the first things that strikes us about this case is the clear statement of Scripture, confirming an observation which has been made repeatedly in this book, that *sin is not necessarily a cause of childlessness.* The parties in this marriage *"were both righteous before God"* and were "walking in all the commandments and ordinances of the Lord *blameless."* They were blameless! Therefore sin was neither a precipitating nor contributing cause of childlessness in the case of Elisabeth and Zacharias.

However, in spite of their righteousness, they still had a double-edged problem: Elisabeth was barren and on top of that, both she and Zacharias were now "well stricken in years." They were both too old to have children. Their situation was doubly impossible, but *impossibility is no problem for God!*

God's timing is perfect. He arranged for the lot [selection of priests was made by 'chance' through 'the casting of lots'] to fall to Zacharias so that he might be alone burning incense at the altar of the Lord. There he was met by the angel, Gabriel, who explained the reason for his presence: "... Fear not, Zacharias: for thy prayer is heard; and thy wife Elisabeth shall bear thee a son, and thou shalt call his name John." (1:13)

Significantly the angel joined Zacharias at the altar of incense, the place of offering up sweet-smelling savor to God. The incense is a figure for the prayers of the saints, and is typical of Communication with God. It is at the altar of incense that God would speak or answer man!

The message spoken is extremely enlightening. He first told Zacharias who was fearful, not to fear (there is no need to). Then he said thy prayer [petition, *singular*] has been heard. (My personal feeling is that this means that the very first prayer on the subject that Zacharias prayed was heard.) The angel also is informing us that the specific key to victory over childlessness in this case was the fervent *prayer prayed by Zacharias.* This also reminds us of the prayers prayed by Isaac, Leah, Rachael, and Hannah. Then pre-natal instructions were given to permit John to be a Nazarite from birth, and to be filled with the Holy Spirit even before his birth.

Zacharias like so many before him, doubted when the promise was given. He asked how he could know for sure the truth of the promise, because of the weight of the natural evidence to the contrary: "I am an old man, and my wife is well stricken in years." Gentlemanly, and humanly he focused his doubt primarily upon his own inadequacy.

Gabriel responded by identifying himself, as "Gabriel, that stand in the presence of God; and am sent to speak unto thee, and to show thee these glad tidings." (1:19) He had been sent right from the very Throne of God to answer Zacharias's prayer and to arrange the details for his son's birth.

"And, behold, thou shalt be dumb, and not able to speak, until the day that these things shall be performed, because thou believest not my words, which shall be fulfilled in their season." (1:20)

He asked the angel to prove or confirm the promise with a sign. He got a sign as an assurance, but it was not what he had expected, I'm sure! Because of the doubt manifested by Zacharias, he was struck dumb in accordance with another portion of the angel's prophecy. He became unable to speak for a season, until the miracle was performed and the prophecy fulfilled. The very inability to speak not only confirmed the availability of the power to perform the other miracle, but also prevented him from speaking any further doubt, until the fact of the birth was established.

Note carefully however, that Zacharias's doubt did not prevent nor frustrate the plans, purposes, nor even the timing of God. It did not delay for even one moment God's timetable. He was dumb, unable to speak for probably about ten or eleven months (estimating one month to complete his period of service and to return home, plus the nine month gestation period, and the eight days until the circumcision of the child).

We have noted the reasons for the dumbness, but what was its effect upon him, why did God choose to punish his doubt with silence? Zacharias couldn't fully enjoy the forthcoming event. He couldn't go out with his friends and say, "Oh, by the way, did I mention that I'm about to become a father?" He forfeited some of the joy, that otherwise might have been his. This childless man in his old age, couldn't rejoice vocally in advance of the fact, but he did afterwards! (1:64)

Elisabeth conceived. The miracle occurs and she exalts as so many of the other women we have considered, "Thus hath the Lord dealt with me in the days wherein he looked on me, to take away my reproach among men." (1:25)

We also find one of the most beautiful miracle promises concerning the conception of a child, spoken by Gabriel in connection with Elisabeth: "And, behold, thy cousin Elisabeth, she hath also conceived a son in her old age: and this is the sixth month with her, who was called barren. *For with God nothing shall be impossible.*" (1:36,37)

Elisabeth received the blessing of a son in her old age, as

the result of the fervent prayer of her righteous husband. The birth of her son was a great source of joy to her and her neighbors and cousins heard of it and the joined her in rejoicing. (1:57) Both she and Zacharias were faithful and obedient to the instructions received and did name their newborn son, "John." Their obedience was rewarded, and both were enabled to give utterances under the anointing of the Holy Ghost.

9. Truths From Mary - *Favor Found*
Matthew 1, Luke 1 & 2

"Now the birth of Jesus Christ was on this wise: When as his mother Mary was espoused to Joseph, before they came together, she was found with child of the Holy Ghost." (Matt. 1:18)

In the account of Mary we find the greatest miracle birth ever recorded, that of a virgin who was enabled to conceive a son without the aid of a male partner. Truly nothing is too difficult for, nor beyond the ability of, our God!

Gabriel arrives and tells her to fear not, removing a source of stress for her. It is helpful to get rid of all fears, especially of those that would tend to cause doubt or unbelief concerning conception. He also advises her of the reason for her blessedness: she has found favor [grace = unmerited favor] with God. He gives her the promise and encourages her faith for the seemingly impossible by, in effect, giving her a testimony. He tells her of the experience of her cousin, Elisabeth, who had been barren but was by then six months along.

Mary responds to Gabriel's prophetic promise with beautiful simplicity of obedience and of acceptance. She received further encouragement to her faith when her cousin, under the anointing of the Holy Ghost prophesied to her, addressing her as "the mother of my Lord." The angel also gave confirmation to Joseph in a dream to encourage him to accept the fact of a wife-to-be who was with child. (Matt. 1:20) The couple then continued faithfully serving the Lord and journeyed to Bethlehem where the promise was fulfilled in the birth of Jesus.

God gave to mankind the greatest love gift ever given. God's greatest gift came, wrapped not in swaddling clothes, but in human flesh, the gift of His own Son. By that same act, he restored to fallen mankind - the *tree of life* - wrapped not in bark, but rather, in the human flesh of his own son.

* * * * *

Eve was not mentioned in our listing of barren women, but in a certain sense we probably should add Eve to our list of supernatural conceptions. Even though the birth that she experienced was natural in retrospect, at the time no one had ever before conceived.

For Eve it was a first time occurrence. For the world it was a first time occurrence. It was something new, it was something different. If I were to hold up a piece of paper, and lightning came down and struck the paper setting it afire, it would be a natural function, because lightning can cause fire. But, even though it was a natural occurrence, it still would be miraculous to us, because we've never seen it happen before. In that sense, the conception and birth that Eve experienced, were supernatural. It was the first time conception or birth had ever happened. Even though we accept it as normal, childbearing was a new thing. When it happened for Eve, it had never happened before.

B. PRAYER WORKS: MODERN EXAMPLES

1. Wilma and Nelson

Shortly after Sue and I were baptized in the Holy Spirit, we had an opportunity to share about our experiences with a young couple who happened to be unable to have children. We explained the salvation message with them from a tract, because we were then very inexperienced. They prayed with us to accept Jesus as their Lord and Saviour. They then suggested that we might pray for them to be able to have a child. The doctors had told them that they were "medically allergic" to one another (she was apparently producing anti-sperm antibodies), that for some inexplicable reason her body was destroying his sperm, and that "there was no possible way for them to have children naturally." This had been the final determination after almost five years and attempting to remedy the problem with a variety of drug therapies. So we did agree with them in prayer for God to bless them with a baby.

A month or so later while out of town on a business trip, the husband was praying and the Lord quickened to him a passage of Scripture that he had read earlier that morning, from Psalm 113:9, "He maketh the barren woman to keep house, and to be a joyful mother of children." Nelson called us to share the exciting news that he felt God had 'spoken to him' in giving him that Scriptural promise, and that he was now sure that God was going to give them a child.

For the next thirty days, he continued to stand upon that promise and on the thirtieth day they later learned, his wife Wilma did indeed conceive their first son. She, who had been diagnosed by the best doctors available to be "permanently infertile," would later have two more sons and a daughter. I am convinced, as they are, that their children came as a direct result of prayer and of the intervention of God.

God often does more than we expect in answering prayer. He did so in this case. He not only gave them more children than they had anticipated, but He also taught them to trust in Him, to know Him as an Answerer of prayer, revealed Himself as a miracle-working God, and gave them a testimony of His faithfulness to share with others.

2. Charlene and Ed

Another couple of very dear friends, Ed and Charlene, had an almost identical situation. After having sought medical assistance, for their infertility and being told by three different doctors that "there was no way they could ever have children." they were despairing. We shared with them the 'good news' of my having found a miracle-working God, who had healed me of terminal cancer after the doctors had given up on me. They believed the truth and decided to ask us to agree with them in prayer for the healing of their infertility problem. (We didn't yet know at this point about the answer to Nelson and Wilma's prayer.)

Ed told me years later that he, too, had been out of town on a business trip, and decided in his desperation to pray again for Charlene. He laughed as he related the details, "I was in my hotel room seventeen stories up, with no nearby buildings nearly as high. Nonetheless, as a baby Christian, I carefully closed the shades, knelt down alongside the bed, folded my hands and prayed as sincerely as I knew how. Would you believe it," he continued, "God gave me that passage from Psalm 113 about 'the barren woman being the joyful mother of a houseful of children.'"

"I really felt that something significant had happened, in that hotel room; and so on the way home, I stopped at an airport shop and bought a stuffed toy animal. I handed it to Charlene when I got home and told her that she was going to have a baby. She looked at me like she thought I was 'nuts.' But when I explained what had happened to me when I had prayed in the hotel room, she and I both then got down on our knees and prayed together for a child. In less than three months she had conceived, and nine months later delivered a healthy son. Two years later we again prayed, asking God to do another miracle, and He did. We had a daughter. The Ob/Gyn who had tested Charlene originally, delivered both of our children and he 'nearly dropped his teeth' each time when she went to him and tested pregnant. He couldn't believe it!" Ed concluded with a grin.

3. Fertility Power

A further testimonial to the potential 'fertility power' in that passage was provided when Dr. Ritter shared with me the case of a woman who had come from another part of the state to see him. The lady had blocked Fallopian tubes which would have required surgery if she were to be treated. He mentioned the promise of Psalm 113:9 to her and prayed with her before she left to consider her options. He later received a letter from her, thanking him for visiting with her, and advising him that she was already pregnant (without medical treatment)!

It is important to point out that Psalm 113:9 is not a magic wand nor an "open sesame" that will always result in conception. Obviously it does not, fortunately, have the same effect upon each individual who reads it. But it can function as a trigger for faith for those who are seeking God for a child, as can any other Scripture which the Lord may choose to 'quicken' to you. Any verse that causes faith to rise in your heart, or your faith to be built that God can and will do miraculous things, can function in the same way for you.

4. Jan and Bob

Jan came to my prayer room and said, "I'd like to have you pray for me, that I might be able to have children. The Lord blessed me when I was here the last time, when I received the baptism in the Holy Spirit, and now I'd like prayer that my husband and I might be able to have children. We have been unable, and have already been the medical route. The doctors have said that it is impossible for us to have children."

Jan then continued, "We have attempted unsuccessfully to conceive for over a year. We have gone the medical route. I went to a doctor whose name was supernaturally given to me: I heard his name brought up in conversations three times within two days, and later found out he was a Christian. On that basis, I decided he was the doctor I wanted to go to. He tested me, did all the normal things, performed all the standard tests on me. Then he and his his staff tested both my husband and me, and found that the tests were normal. His sperm count was normal, and there was no physical indication of any problem within myself."

"When he tested me," she explained, "He said he saw nothing wrong. However, after the tests, he asked, 'Would you mind if I prayed for you?' He then prayed that we might be blessed with children. Afterwards, he pulled out his Bible and read a couple of promises about childbearing."

"On a subsequent visit to his office after I had made love with my husband earlier that morning, the doctor was able to recover sperm in a sample from my body, and found that it was all dead. Somehow, some kind of strange process was taking place within us, and my body chemistry was killing my husband's sperm cells. Each of us, individually, was okay but together we were 'poison.' Apparently it had to do with the PH factor in my body chemistry my acidity was reacting with his alkaline factor, or something of the sort. This was a phenomenon they acknowledged to be very rare, so they took blood tests, packed the blood samples in dry ice and sent them to Oregon, which is one of the few places in the country where they can test for this particular type of problem."

"Meanwhile, my husband had been referred to a urologist who said, after he'd seen the results, 'We never say never, because there are things that we don't understand that sometimes happen. However, based on the findings, you have a real problem and it's highly unlikely that you would ever be able to conceive regardless of the type of treatment we were to give you.' They called a clinic in New York, because this condition was so rare, that apparently there are only about a dozen cases in the entire country. The urologist there did say that there might be a slim chance. The New York clinic had been able to help one individual in one instance by treating with steroids, although of course, they warned, there are side effects."

"I'd also like to have Bob come and see you for prayer." Jan said slightly desperately. Bob, a young man with a very sweet spirit, came a few days later desiring the Baptism in the Spirit. Afterwards, he eagerly agreed with me in prayer for the healing of their infertility problem.

Jan returned a few months later and brought me up to date. "The next week after Bob was here, we went to our weekly prayer group, and had them pray also for us to be able to have children. About a month later the impossible happened and I conceived."

They now have three beautiful children and continue to walk with the Lord.

5. Alice and Ted

Alice came to see me crushed with disappointment, "I've just got to have prayer or I'll go crazy." She blurted out. "We have been trying to have a baby for three years or more now without even a glimmer of hope from the doctors, and now this ... " Her voice trailed off.

"What is it that's happened now, to make the situation worse?" I asked.

"Ted has just gotten the results of his most recent sperm test. I think this was the one they said measured motility." She sobbed, "And the doctor said he'd never even heard of a count as low as Ted's. He said his was about 1 or 2. Normal should be something over 100,000,000. He said, he didn't want to be unkind, but that we were wasting our time and money seeking help. I appreciate his honesty, but ... "

I attempted to comfort her, and reminded her that "nothing is too difficult for the Lord: He can do all things!" I also pointed out that even one sperm was sufficient, technically, to get the job done. I then shared with her some of the promises for fertility in the Scripture and simply suggested that we pray in faith, to give God an opportunity to demonstrate His miracle working power and provision in her behalf.

I think Alice was one of the most beautiful pregnant women I have ever seen. She was radiant and bore a broad smile every time that I saw her during her pregnancy. She and Ted have had three children and continue to witness to God's miracle working power.

6. Callie and Randy

Callie was, or rather is, a beautiful young woman who came to visit me for ministry long before the matter of child-lessness was a concern for her. She received various ministry over the years including the Baptism in the Holy Spirit and deliverance from several extensive spirit groups that had greatly hindered her, including a major alcohol addiction. When she married, she became concerned as to whether or not she would be able to conceive. A doctor had told her while she was till a teen that due to her having a tilted womb and certain other structural problems, she would have a difficult time becoming pregnant if she were ever able to. He also warned that she would probably not be able to carry a child to term, or to have a normal healthy child.

Callie and Randy both turned to the Lord before they were

112

married and both were Baptized in the Spirit. Callie had a physical shortly before and said the doctors were amazed at how her body apparently had not been at all affected by her addiction or the previous physical problems for which we had prayed and God had healed.

Interestingly, Callie and Randy were able to conceive within a few months of their marriage and she has also had subsequent children. Callie called me from the hospital recovery room to tell me she'd just had her first baby. She was ecstatic, as well she should have been, for God had miraculously blessed her with her first, perfect, healthy, miracle baby.

The next phase is to step out in faith...

PART V

PUTTING FAITH INTO ACTION

"But without faith it is impossible to please him:
for he that cometh to God must believe
that *he is*, and that he *is a rewarder*
of them that diligently seek him."
(Heb. 11:6)

PART V

PUTTING FAITH INTO ACTION

A. HOW DO WE GET FAITH?

The word of God tells us that "faith cometh by hearing and hearing by the word of God." So, finding a relevant promise in the Scripture or hearing a modern testimony can build faith. Jesus, Himself, specifically encouraged the faith of a parent in regard to the healing of an afflicted offspring whose very life was being threatened, when he gave a similar unlimited promise to the father of the epileptic boy:

> "Jesus said unto him, If thou canst believe, *all things are possible* to him that believeth."
> (Mk. 9:23)

It is thus clear to any reader of the Scripture that God promises unlimited results to those who can believe, or who can utilize faith. Therefore, it certainly behooves us to understand what faith is. The Scripture defines it and gives a boost to our faith in a passage written by Paul to the Hebrews:

> "But without faith it is impossible to please him: for he that cometh to God must believe that *he is,* and that he *is a rewarder* of them that diligently seek him." (Heb. 11:6)

At first this seems difficult, but as we meditate upon this

117

passage, we see blessed truth! First we see that it is indeed impossible to please God without faith, but we know that faith is a "gift ... lest any man boast." (Eph 2:8,9) Second, we see that the faith required to please God is very simple: we must believe *that God exists* [is], and that *He does reward those who diligently seek Him.* That doesn't seem too hard, I think even I can believe that. Thus basic, God-pleasing faith is simple.

It must not require a great quantity of faith even to work miracles, for Jesus also said unto them, "Because of your unbelief: for verily I say unto you, If ye have faith as a grain of mustard seed, ye shall say unto this mountain, Remove hence to yonder place; and it shall remove; and *nothing shall be impossible unto you.*" (Mat. 17:20)

Faith, when you come right down to it, cannot be that difficult. Think of all the simple, uneducated men and women in the Scriptural accounts who pleased God with their faith. Many who were praised for great faith didn't even have the benefit of an acquaintance with the Law, Jewish teaching or tradition. Consider the Centurion whose faith Jesus praised.[1]

The point to be clearly established is that faith - even great faith - is attainable! It consists in simply believing the Word of God to be true; the promises of God in His Word to be true, and then in relying upon them and obeying (the Word of God) in spite of all seeming evidence to the contrary. Jonah from the belly of the whale, in the vilest of circumstances with the weeds wrapped about his head, spoke from a heart filled with faith when he said, "They that observe *lying vanities* forsake their own mercy ... I will pay that I have vowed. *Salvation is of the LORD.*" (Jonah 2:8,9b) The Lord responded to his statement of faith, and spoke unto the fish, "and it vomited out Jonah upon the dry land." Jonah by faith perceived that his

----

1. Matthew. 8:5ff

118

own circumstances were "lying vanities" and that, in spite of them, his Lord was a saving God: a Saviour!

Jesus offered to us another tremendous encouragement- to-believe promise when He told His disciples, speaking in regard to salvation,

"But Jesus beheld them, and said unto them, With men this is impossible; but with God *all things are possible.*" (Mat. 19:26)

The Scripture makes it abundantly clear that faith is attainable, and tells us three specific ways that faith can be increased:

1.) by **hearing the Word of God:**
"So then faith cometh by hearing, and hearing by the word of God." (Rom. 10:17)

2.) by **praying in the Spirit:**
"But ye, beloved, building up yourselves on your most holy faith, praying in the Holy Ghost." (Jude 1:20) and,

3.) by **hearing a testimony:**
"And they overcame him by the blood of the Lamb, and by the word of their testimony; and they loved not their lives unto the death." (Rev. 12:11)

Thus, faith can be established in a believer's heart by hearing (or reading) the Word of God, and having that Word energized within His spirit by the Holy Spirit; or, by praying in the Holy Spirit. Through giving himself completely to the will of the Spirit and determining to cooperate with, and yeild to, the Spirit, the believer finds his faith being built up. Finally, the faith to be victorious against the wiles of the devil and to overcome, or defeat, him comes as a result of the believer utilizing (applying in faith) the Blood of the Lamb, by speaking the words of his testimony, and by being willing to risk his own life for the sake of the Kingdom.

The word of one individual's testimony to the faithfulness of Jesus to answer prayer, or to fulfill one of the promises of Scripture, builds faith for the hearer himself to believe God for the same kind of miraculous fulfillment. It stimulates belief by confirming both the faithfulness and the veracity of the Word of God. It blesses and strengthens us to hear of others who have placed their trust in God and found He answered their prayers or met their needs. It thus encourages us to likewise dare to trust in Him.

A FORMULA FOR FAITH

It is imperative to know *what* the will of God is concerning the matter for which you desire to have faith. You may say, "I know that God is able to heal; I have complete faith that He can heal me!" But, TO KNOW THAT GOD *CAN HEAL*, DOES NOT CONSTITUTE *FAITH* THAT HE *WILL HEAL!*

An illustration might help: I believe with all my heart that the president of our local bank can write me a check for $100,000.00. I don't have the slightest doubt in his *ability* to do it. However, I must confess to you that I have absolutely *zero faith* that he will write me such a check! Therefore to know that someone can do something is not enough to create faith that they will do it. Thus, there is a missing ingredient that must be added to our knowledge of the person's ability to do the thing needed; we *MUST* also know that it is *the will* (the desire, the intent) of that person to do the thing that we are trying to muster faith for: in this case, for our healing from childlessness. WE *MUST* KNOW GOD'S WILL!

Years ago while seeking my own healing from terminal cancer, the Lord quickened this truth to me in an almost formula-like statement, "IT IS IMPOSSIBLE TO HAVE FAITH IN

GOD TO DO ANYTHING THAT WE DO NOT KNOW TO
BE THE WILL OF GOD!" Let that truth sink in: let God burn
it down into your heart, for it is a key to truth and victory in
Him! Without this as a foundation for our faith, we are just
going through the motions.

It may be easier to grasp this truth if stated negatively: "It
Is Impossible To Have Faith In God To Do Anything, That We
Think God *Doesn't Want* To Do!"

It is therefore essential, if FAITH for the healing of our
situation is to exist, that we KNOW WHAT GOD'S WILL IS
REGARDING the MATTER OF *CHILDLESSNESS!*

I found it fairly easy to believe for someone else to be
healed. Sure, the promises of healing in the Scriptures were
quite clear, but my burning question was, "What about *me?*
Did God want to heal me?"

I found the answer to that question as I had the answers to
all my other questions, in the Word of God. The answer I
found is in the fifth chapter of Luke, in Jesus's own words!

A certain leper approached Jesus and said to Him, "Lord if
thou wilt, thou canst make me clean."[1] What the leper was
really saying was, "Lord, if it was your *will to* do it, you could
make me clean and whole of my leprosy."

Jesus answered the question of that leper, and my question
as well, when He responded with a touch of His hand and said,
"*I will*; be thou clean." and the leper was immediately made
whole.

Jesus, in essence, said to the leper, (and to me, and to

----

1. Luke 5:12,13

121

you): "I *DO WILL IT*, IT IS MY WILL ... MY DESIRE ...
MY INTENT ... BE THOU MADE WHOLE!" [1]

Thus, in order for you to have real faith that you will have
a child, there are certain questions for which you must find
answers:

    1.) Is it the will of God for His followers to have
children, if they desire to have them?

    2.) Are children a blessing? (see Part II)

    3.) Is it the will of God *for you* to have a child?

    4.) Is it God's will *to heal you*, if necessary, so that
you can have children? [2]

With these matters settled in your heart, you can indeed
have faith for God to bless you with a child.

However, it is essential to remember that God is sovereign
and that both His planning and His timing are perfect. One
truth that I have often shared in teaching sessions, and have
frequently been told brought help to the hearers, is to remember that *A DELAY IS NOT A NO!* Just because we do not have
the object of our desire in hand, does not mean that it is not
enroute!

Everyone who finds himself confronted with the task of
praying for something, usually at some point find himself
wondering, "Do I have enough faith?" The issue of faith and of
how to attain faith are important and worthy of consideration.
As we approach the issue from the viewpoint of desiring to
overcome barrenness we realize that we need to settle for

----

1. For a more comprehensive consideration of the issue of healing, and of God's will
to heal, see the book *Alive Again!* by the same author.

2. If you still have doubt in this area, we suggest you read the chapter, "Is It God's
Will To Heal *You*?" in *Alive Again!* by the same author.

ourselves certain important issues.

B. HOW TO PRAY

An important question that should be prayerfully considered by any Christian couple confronted with the problem of childlessness is, "What part does God play in the solution being pursued? Could the healing that's being sought, be accomplished (by means of medicine, surgery, or an in-vitro solution) if there were no God?" Specific prayer for being blessed with children puts God in the equation, recognizes Him as all-powerful, acknowledges Him as the source of life, and potentially gives Him honor when the pregnancy or birth occurs.

1. Praying The Word

It is tremendously faith-inspiring for me when I can find specific instances in Scripture where God dealt with the very same type of problem that I am seeking to overcome. This is certainly true with healing or deliverance. If I am having a problem with a bad knee, my faith is increased, for example, when I see one of His promises such as:

> "Strengthen ye the weak hands, and confirm [make firm] the feeble *knees*." (Isa. 35:3)

or,

> "I *will walk* before the LORD in the land of the living." (Psa. 116:9)

So, too, when a need for fertility or conception exists, if a promise can be found that relates to being fertile or to conceiving, or if an instance of that problem being overcome by prayer or the intervention of God is discovered, then faith is encouraged. Faith for conception, child-bearing, healthy delivery and for the healing of unhealthy babies or children will be built up in this chapter as we consider cases recorded in the Scriptures, and modern testimonies.

"Shall I bring to the birth, and not cause to bring forth? saith the LORD: shall I cause to bring forth, and shut the womb? saith thy God." (Isa. 66:9)

2. Prayer Plus The Word Is A Powerful Force

Joan's Endometriosis & Perseverance

Recently, at a meeting, an attractive young woman came up to me and asked, "Aren't you, Mr. Banks?"

I responded, "Yes, I am. Although your face is familiar, I'm afraid I don't recall your name."

"It's Joan Miller, but I wouldn't expect you to remember my name, but I certainly do remember you!" She replied emphatically. "I met you on January twenty-first of 1983. I came into your bookstore and spoke with your wife at the counter and she said, 'You need to talk with my husband.' She then led me back to your prayer room ... and I was born again at 12:00 noon on the twenty-first of January, 1983."

"You probably don't recall it, but I also received a great healing miracle from the Lord. I was struggling desperately years ago to have a child, but the doctors told me it was impossible for me to conceive a child. I had endometriosis," She explained, "When I was told I couldn't have a child, I refused to believe it."

"I sought one medical opinion after another, until six doctors had all told me the same thing, and it finally sank in. However, I still refused to accept the medical diagnosis, because I believed God was bigger than my problem, and that He could certainly heal me of endometriosis or of anything else that would prevent me having a child. I found scriptural promises concerning fruitfulness and healing, and I continued to seek him wholeheartedly for my healing."

Joan's face seemed to glow, as she concluded her brief testimony, "God did it! He healed me! I not only conceived, but I now have three children!"

Joan's account reminds us of a particularly significant fact: there is a need to continue seeking the Lord, wholeheartedly, with perseverance, remembering that "Nothing is too difficult for our God!" This latter truth is clearly brought out in the Scripture, in a promise passage spoken by an angel that has to do specifically with a birth that would have been impossible without the direct intervention of God, by His Spirit:

"For with God nothing shall be impossible."
(Luk. 1:37)

"He maketh the barren woman to keep house, and to be a joyful mother of children. Praise ye the Lord." (Psa. 113:9)

"Sing, O barren, thou that didst not bear; break forth into singing, and cry aloud, thou that didst not travail with child: for more are the children of the desolate than the children of the married wife, saith the LORD." (Isa. 54:1)

The two scriptures above have had a powerful impact upon the lives of many formerly childless couples. The first is a favorite of Dr. Ritter's who wrote the foreword. While in private practice he often shared it with patients who were having trouble conceiving. God, it seems, frequently desires to give those seeking Him, a tangible promise from the Scripture to be able to focus their faith upon. He did this with the first Scripture above for Nelson and Wilma, whose acount we considered in the last chapter.

Therefore, read the Word of God *expecting* Him to speak to you through it. He may give you a special word through a passage that doesn't mean anything to anyone else ... but does have a special meaning for you, personally!

3. Be Willing To Seek Deliverance?

There is a valid need for the ministry of deliverance in the body of Christ today, perhaps as never before. It has been truthfully stated, "You cannot deliver the flesh"; and by the same token, one cannot crucify a demon! *The flesh must be crucified and demons must be cast out.*

Deliverance is, of course, the casting out of evil spirits, or demons, a subject which seems very foreign to us in our modern, sophisticated society, but it was an area of ministry in which Jesus engaged. In fact, approximately one-fourth of His earthly ministry was devoted to dealing with demonic problems and the casting out of demons. Jesus cast out spirits of *infirmity* (Luke 13:11), of *blindness* (Matthew 12:22), spirits causing *speech problems* (Luke 11:14), causing *torment* (Matthew 15:22), causing *aberrational behavior* (Luke 8:27), and causing *suicidal behavior* (Mark 9:22), to mention but a few. This deliverance ministry wasn't limited to Jesus alone, but rather was something which He commissioned those who followed Him to also make available. (Mark 16:17, Matthew 10:8)

We find the followers of Jesus also engaging in this ministry of deliverance, as the ministry of the "pattern evangelist" Philip bears testimony. We can observe his ministry in Samaria (Acts 8:7), where "unclean spirits crying with loud voice came out of many that were possessed with them." Paul also ministered deliverance when an occult *spirit of divination* to a young girl who was following after him and Silas (Acts 16:18).

We have provided simple prayers in this book to enable you to deal with the spiritual problems which may be encountered. However, if you feel the need do not hesitate to seek out a mature prayer partner or counselor to help you.

126

4. The Proper Prayer of Faith

The first two couples with whom we prayed after ourselves receiving the baptism of the Holy Spirit, after we had shared salvation and the truths of the baptism of the Holy Spirit with them, shared with us that they had been trying unsuccessfully to have children. They then asked if we would pray that they might be able to have a child. The two couples have subsequently had a total of six children born to them. Both had been diagnosed as medically incompatible, and been told that it would "be impossible for them to conceive."

These births confirm the next point we wish to observe, that very frequently, the blessings of children are delayed until prayer is properly offered. Before you leave me in disgust, let me explain what I mean by "proper" prayer. I am not referring to proper wording of a prayer, but rather to *that prayer which the Lord requires or desires.* Most of us, if we are honest, will admit that we would prefer to have our prayers answered at home, in the privacy of our bedroom or prayer closet. This is certainly true of our prayers for healing in general, and especially in the case of a more private and personal need such as that of conception. However, God's plan, as outlined in the Bible, includes certain provisions that He has made, such as, gifts of healing, (1 Cor. 12:9); and the specific provision for the sick Christian in James 5:14ff, of seeking prayer from the elders.

Having conducted hundreds of healing services over the past nineteen years, I've often encountered reluctant "prayees" who often ask this very question, "Why did I have to come forward in a meeting to be healed? Why couldn't God have healed me at home without all of this?" The "this," referring apparently to the embarrassment of having to make their need known publicly and to humble themselves by submitting to prayer from others in the body.

My usual response is, "God certainly could have healed

you at home, but for His purposes, He obviously hasn't yet chosen to do so. Thus, He has caused you to seek prayer here, perhaps for one of these reasons: to humble yourself to submit to prayer, to show you how the body was intended to function, to show you how the gifts of the spirit were intended to operate, to teach you and those of us present to depend, or rely upon the body. Also through you He is giving the body an opportunity to minister; an opportunity for someone else's faith to be built by seeing you healed; and perhaps even creating a situation to encourage someone else to come forward."

Thus, we can see that a "proper prayer" is *a prayer offered in accordance with the will of God for you by that individual or those individuals whom the Lord wishes to use in lifting that need to Himself.*

We have seen that the natural part of receiving a miracle includes a combination of building up of our own faith through prayer and study, and seeking the prayers of the Body of Christ. Now, having "done all" we can on our part to become righteous, it is time to stand in faith awaiting the promise, but first one more word of encouragement and of testimony....

PART VI

A FINAL WORD

"I am the vine, ye are the branches: He that abideth in me, and I in him, the same bringeth forth much fruit: for without me ye can do nothing." (John 15:5)

PART VI

A FINAL WORD

A TESTIMONY TO PAINLESS CHILDBIRTH

A young woman, a close Christian friend, came to my prayer room one afternoon, and said, "I want to share something with you. Actually, I want to get your opinion on something I've come to see in the Scripture."

I knew that Pam and her husband, John, had both experienced healings, some rather dramatic, were both saved and had been baptized in the Holy Spirit. She continued, "We know from Galatians that Jesus became a curse for us that we might be freed from the curse, right?"

"True." I agreed.

"Since I've become pregnant, we've been looking for scriptures concerning pregnancy, and Genesis 3:16 makes it clear, the curse placed upon Eve included pain in childbearing. I believe that Jesus paid the price for that curse as well as He did for all the other curses; therefore, I shouldn't have to undergo any pain in childbirth. And, I want to have my baby at home."

I liked the concept, but had to confess that it had never occurred to me, and so I told her, "Theologically, what you say makes sense. However, I have to be honest and confess to you, I don't know that I would have the faith to stand on that premise, to believe that there will be no pain in childbearing, and would want to have the baby at home as you've expressed to be your desire. But, it certainly sounds right."

With confidence in what God had shown her, Pam subsequently had three children, all basically delivered at home by her husband. The confirmation of what the Lord had shown to them was the lack of pain in all three deliveries. Her first delivery was very long, as the first often is, but she experienced no contractions that were painful. She told me later, that not once did she have to stifle a cry from pain.

The second child was delivered in their bathroom after sampling too many of the chocolate chip cookies which she'd made the day previous to the birth. She awoke that night with gas problems, and a tightness in her abdomen. The gas brought on labor, again without pain, but with extreme relief from the gas. The baby delivered with no pain and so quickly that her husband barely had time to get to her to catch the baby. Her second and third babies were each born in one hour's time.

God's provision is perfect in every instance. Still, it is important for us to hear the "word of testimony" because such often enable us to believe or trust God for more than we could have, without having our own faith stimulated by the faith enhancing accounts. Pam's testimony should be a real faith builder for those who are facing labor, as well for others who just need to have their faith stretched. Several women have shared with me that my relating Pam's experience to them helped build their faith to ask God for their own painless deliveries.

We need to have our concept of God's ability expanded. Far too many of us are hindered by such limitation as the Scripture states in James 4:2b, "Ye have not because ye ask not."

* * * * *

I have been doubly blessed in being permitted to have the privilege of conducting services for, and dedicating to the Lord, some of the miracle babies whose stories have been related in this book. Their very existence as well as each of their lives remain a testimonial to His faithfulness and miracle working power. Remember that *all conception and every birth is miraculous.*

Our Scriptural prayer for you, if you are seeking children remains: "Be fruitful and multiply ..." (Gen. 1:28) and that you might find victory over, and *deliverance from, childlessness!*

Editor's Note:

We trust that this book has been a blessing to you. If you feel that it has helped you, and especially if you are helped in having a child, feel free to write the author, or to send a photograph, in care of

IMPACT BOOKS, INC.
137 W. Jefferson,
Kirkwood, Mo. 63122

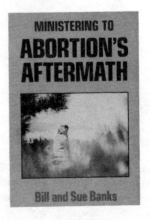

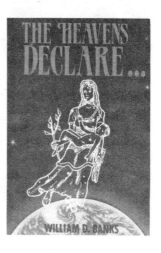
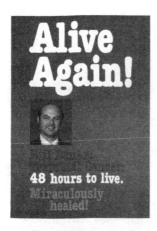

FOR ADDITIONAL COPIES WRITE:

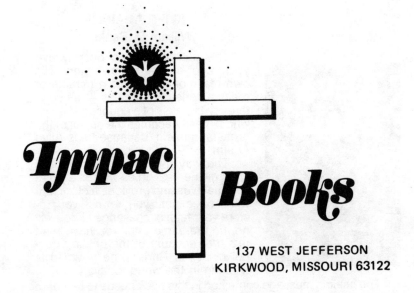

Impac Books

137 WEST JEFFERSON
KIRKWOOD, MISSOURI 63122